Pharmacology

FOR TECHNICIANS

Don A. Ballington
Mary M. Laughlin
Skye A. McKennon

Sixth Edition

Workbook

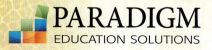

PARADIGM
EDUCATION SOLUTIONS

St. Paul

Senior Vice President	Linda Hein
Managing Editor	Brenda M. Palo
Developmental Editor	Stephanie Schempp
Director of Production	Timothy W. Larson
Production Editor	Carrie Rogers
Copyeditor	Suzanne Clinton
Proofreader	Margaret Trejo
Cover and Text Designer	Dasha Wagner
Layout Designer	Jaana Bykonich
Vice President Sales and Marketing	Scott Burns
Director of Marketing	Lara Weber McLellan
Digital Projects Manager	Tom Modl
Digital Production Manager	Aaron Esnough
Web Developer	Blue Earth Interactive

Care has been taken to verify the accuracy of information presented in this book. However, the authors, editors, and publisher cannot accept responsibility for Web, e-mail, newsgroup, or chat room subject matter or content, or for consequences from application of the information in this book, and make no warranty, expressed or implied, with respect to its content.

Trademarks: Some of the product names and company names included in this book have been used for identification purposes only and may be trademarks or registered trade names of their respective manufacturers and sellers. The authors, editors, and publisher disclaim any affiliation, association, or connection with, or sponsorship or endorsement by, such owners.

We have made every effort to trace the ownership of all copyrighted material and to secure permission from copyright holders. In the event of any question arising as to the use of any material, we will be pleased to make the necessary corrections in future printings. Thanks are due to the authors, publishers, and agents listed in the Photo Credits for permission to use the materials therein indicated.

978-0-76386-784-3 (Text)
978-0-76386-781-2 (eBook)

© 2017 by Paradigm Publishing, Inc., a division of EMC Publishing, LLC
875 Montreal Way
St. Paul, MN 55102
E-mail: educate@emcp.com
Web site: www.emcp.com

Printed in the United States of America

23 22 21 20 19 18   3 4 5 6 7 8 9 10

CONTENTS

PREFACE

This workbook has been prepared to accompany the text *Pharmacology for Technicians, Sixth Edition* by Don A. Ballington, Mary M. Laughlin, and Skye A. McKennon. Used in conjunction with the textbook and the digital resources on Navigator+, this workbook reinforces student learning of drug groups, drug uses and effects, and other drug facts essential to the work of pharmacy technicians.

Correlated with the structure of the textbook, the workbook provides exercises for each of the 17 chapters, which are organized into four units. Instructors may choose to assign all or some of these exercises as homework or as take-home exams. Alternatively, students may use these exercises as an independent method of assessing their comprehension of the content discussed in the *Pharmacology for Technicians* textbook.

Overview of Chapter Exercises and Activities

Workbook exercises for Chapters 1 through 3 focus on the important foundation material presented in Unit 1, specifically the science of pharmacology and the study of pharmacokinetics.

Workbook exercises for the chapters of Units 2, 3, and 4 (Chapters 4–17) include a range of exercises requiring the recall of key information as well as the application of knowledge and critical thinking necessary in the pharmacy workplace. The following exercise types are provided for Chapters 4–17:

- *Reading Drug Labels and Medication Orders* requires students to apply literacy skills and drug-dispensing knowledge.
- *Understanding the Larger Medical Context* asks students to focus on medical issues such as disease states, anatomy and physiology, and drug classes in order to demonstrate an understanding of why certain drugs are prescribed, how they are used, and their pharmacokinetic effects.
- *Dispensing and Storing Drugs* asks students to identify storage requirements and auxiliary labels necessary to ensure patient safety and compliance.

- *Putting Safety First* expands on safety issues emphasized in the text by asking students to compare presented doses with standard or typical doses in order to recognize potential errors as well as to identify potential drug interactions.
- *Understanding Concepts* encourages students to explore drug classifications, types of medications and their applicability to disease states, and other issues critical to the work of a pharmacy technician.

All workbook chapters also contain one or more sets of matching questions that help students build their vocabulary related to the field of pharmacology.

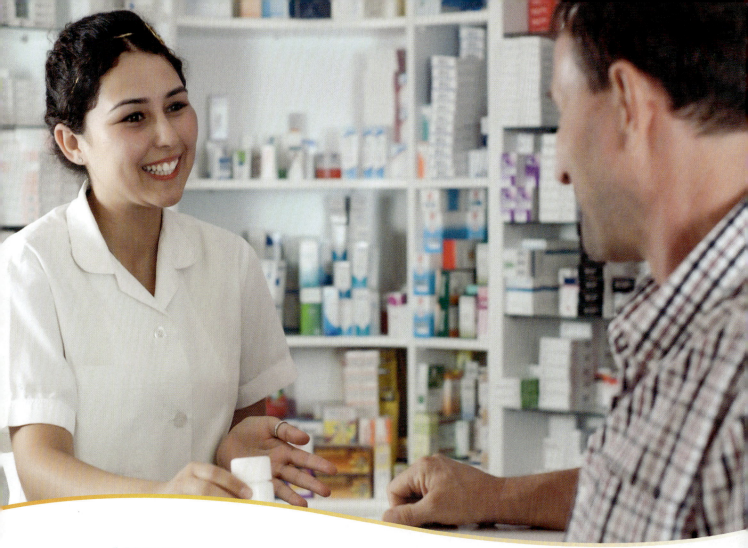

Introduction to Pharmacology

1

Evolution of Medicinal Drugs

Understanding Pharmacology and Pharmacokinetics

1. A company plans to market a new antiseptic solution that prevents the spread of disease on hands and surgical equipment. The marketing department wants to name the product based on a pioneer in the field of chemical sterilization. What two pioneers would you choose? Explain your answer.

   _____

   _____

   _____

2. You are applying for a pharmacy technician job at a retail pharmacy in another state. In the job description, you note the following tasks:
   a. transferring prescriptions
   b. preparing prescription labels
   c. maintaining allergy information in the pharmacy system
   d. counseling diabetics with regard to insulin use

   Which requirements should not be part of the job description?

   _____

   _____

3. What national pharmacy technician association was founded in 1979?

   _____

4. What five organizations formed to make PTCB?

   _____

   _____

Name _____ Date _____

3

5. Put these groups related to pharmaceutical practice in order according to the year of their establishment.

    APhA   USP

    FDA   DEA

    _____

6. You are reading a newspaper advertisement about a drug named BPPA469 for the treatment of osteoarthritis. The advertisement states that healthy adults ages 18 to 45 years are to come in to the clinic once a week to be examined while on BPPA469. What phase of a clinical trial is currently underway with this drug? Explain.

    _____

    _____

7. Which journal (no longer in publication) was the official publication for PTEC?

    _____

8. If you were a student of Galen, what would you consider to be the source of disease?

    _____

9. Name two drug classes that require medication guides to be given to patients at the time they pick up their prescriptions.

    _____

10. Compare and contrast therapeutic and prophylactic drugs.

    _____

    _____

11. During Phase II of a clinical trial, patients are randomized to take either an active drug or a(n) _____.

12. Methotrexate should never be used by pregnant women because of demonstrated harm to the fetus. Using the old categorization, this drug is in FDA pregnancy category _____.

13. A good source for determining whether a generic drug is interchangeable with a brand-name drug is the _____.

14. To be made available without a prescription, a legend drug must have its status changed to _____.

15. To become a credentialed pharmacy technician, an individual must pass a _____ exam.

16. The use of _____ drugs helps to keep the overall cost of healthcare down.

17. Problems with OTC products should be reported to the FDA's _____ or the ISMP.

18. Valerius Cordis published the _____ in 1546.

19. The *Pharmacopoeia of the United States* was first published by the _____.

20. Para-(N-acetyl) aminophenol is an example of a _____ name.

21. Homeopathic remedies use _____ doses of drugs.

22. Each drug seeking marketing status in the United States must have submitted and received an approved _____ .

23. Title II of the Comprehensive Drug Abuse Prevention and Control Act of 1970 designated five schedules for _____ according to the abuse probability of the drugs.

24. Insulin was first isolated by _____ .

25. In a(n) _____ study, neither trial participants nor research staff know which subjects are in the experimental group and which subjects are in the control group.

Matching–Terms and Definitions

_____ 26. A name that identifies a drug independently of its manufacturer; sometimes denotes a drug that is not protected by a trademark; also referred to as a *USAN (United States Adopted Name)*

_____ 27. A government grant that gives a drug company the exclusive right to manufacture a drug for a certain number of years; protects the company's investment in developing the drug

_____ 28. The agency of the US federal government that is responsible for ensuring the safety of drugs and food prepared for the market

_____ 29. The entity, usually a pharmaceutical company, responsible for testing the efficacy and safety of a drug and proposing the drug for approval

_____ 30. The branch of the U.S. Justice Department that is responsible for regulating the sale and use of specified drugs, especially controlled substances

_____ 31. A medicinal substance or remedy used to change the way a living organism functions; also called a *medication*

_____ 32. The form used to order C-II substances

a. black-box warning
b. brand name
c. C-I
d. C-II
e. C-III and C-IV
f. C-V
g. controlled substance
h. drug
i. DEA
j. DEA form 222
k. drug sponsor
l. FDA
m. generic name
n. homeopathy
o. legend drug
p. medication guide
q. OTC drug
r. patent
s. pharmacist
t. pharmacognosy
u. pharmacology
v. pharmacy technician
w. placebo
x. prophylactic drug
y. PTCB

_____ 33. A drug with potential for abuse; organized into five categories or schedules that specify whether and how the drug may be dispensed

_____ 34. A drug with the highest potential for abuse, which may be used only for research under a special license

_____ 35. A drug with a high potential for abuse, for which dispensing is severely restricted and prescriptions may not be refilled

_____ 36. A drug with a moderate potential for abuse, which can be refilled no more than five times in six months and only if authorized by the physician for this time period

_____ 37. A drug with a slight potential for abuse; some of which may be sold without a prescription depending on state law, but the purchaser must sign for the drug and show identification

_____ 38. A drug that may be sold only by prescription and must be labeled "Caution: Federal law prohibits dispensing without prescription" or "Rx only"

_____ 39. Specific information about certain types of drugs that is required by the FDA to be made available to the patient

_____ 40. A drug that may be sold without a prescription

_____ 41. One who is licensed to prepare and sell or dispense drugs and compounds and to fill prescriptions

_____ 42. A drug that prevents or decreases the severity of a disease

_____ 43. An inactive substance with no treatment value

_____ 44. A national organization that develops pharmacy technician standards and serves as a credentialing agency for pharmacy technicians

_____ 45. An individual working in a pharmacy who, under the supervision of a licensed pharmacist, assists in activities not requiring the professional judgment of a pharmacist

_____ 46. The study and identification of natural sources of drugs

_____ 47. The science of drugs and their interactions with the systems of living animals

_____ 48. Information printed on a drug package to alert prescribers to potential problems with the drug

_____ 49. The name under which the manufacturer markets a drug; also known as the _trade name_

_____ 50. A system of therapeutics in which diseases are treated by administering minute doses of drugs that, in healthy patients, are capable of producing symptoms like those of the disease being treated

Basic Concepts of Pharmacology

Understanding Pharmacology and Pharmacokinetics

1. Heart rate increases when beta-1 receptors are stimulated. A drug taken by a patient binds to the beta-1 receptors. As a result, the patient's heart rate increases. Is the drug an antagonist or an agonist? Explain your answer.

   _____

   _____

2. What is the goal of drug therapy?

   _____

   _____

3. Why does the body act to maintain homeostasis?

   _____

4. Ciclopirox (Penlac Nail Lacquer) is an antifungal used to treat onychomycosis, a type of nail fungus. The directions say to apply the lacquer to each affected nail daily. Will the ciclopirox have a local or systemic effect? Explain your answer.

   _____

5. For many cases of infective endocarditis, the combination of gentamicin and ampicillin has been shown to be more effective than using each drug individually. The combination also allows the patient to avoid toxicities associated with the higher doses of gentamicin needed for separate dosing. How would you categorize the relationship of gentamicin and ampicillin when used together?

   _____

6. What are the two types of drug inhibition, and how do they differ?

   _____

   _____

Name _____   Date _____

7. Mrs. Kuchinski, a patient with cancer, has been on high doses of extended-release oxycodone, a narcotic analgesic, for six months to treat her pain. Her medication is being managed by an oncologist. Mrs. Kuchinski does not experience euphoria when taking the prescribed dosage. Is she dependent on or addicted to extended-release oxycodone? Explain your answer.

_____

_____

8. When azithromycin (Z-Pak) is dispensed, the patient is told to take two tablets on the first day, and then one tablet a day until all tablets are gone. What is the purpose of this dosage instruction, and what name is given to the first two tablets?

_____

_____

9. You read in a medical journal about a patient who developed an enlarged liver after taking a drug that has been available for 15 years. Although the enlarged liver can definitely be attributed to the drug, no such reaction has previously been reported. Is the response in this case allergic, anaphylactic, or idiosyncratic?

_____

10. Drug A and drug B are both anticholinergics. To have equal effects, drug A must be dosed six times a day, while drug B is dosed two times a day. Which drug has the longer duration of action? Explain your answer.

_____

_____

11. What is half-life? How many half-lives are needed to eliminate a drug from the body?

_____

_____

12. The _____ prevents many drugs from penetrating the brain.

13. Atorvastatin is a drug used to treat high cholesterol. Do you think atorvastatin has a local effect or a systemic effect? Why? _____.

14. The rate at which a drug is eliminated from a specific volume of blood per unit of time is known as _____.

15. Many older adults or patients who have diabetes experience a condition called *gastroparesis*, which greatly delays gastric emptying time. You would expect that this condition would also delay drug _____.

16. Patients with impaired liver function who take drugs that are not excreted by the kidneys might expect drugs to be present for a _____ amount of time in the blood compared with patients with normal liver function.

17. Drugs that undergo an extensive first-pass effect will have a lower _____ than those drugs that do not.

18. A range of serum concentrations for a particular drug that provides the optimum probability of achieving the desired response with the least probability of toxicity is the _____ .

19. A drug has a blood plasma concentration of 20 mcg/mL. Ten hours later, the plasma concentration is 5 mcg/mL. This drug has a half-life of _____ hours.

Matching–Terms and Definitions

_____ 20. The strength by which a particular chemical messenger binds to its receptor site on a cell

_____ 21. A severe allergic response resulting in immediate, life-threatening respiratory distress, usually followed by vascular collapse and shock and accompanied by hives

_____ 22. Drugs that bind to a receptor site and block the action of the endogenous messenger or other drugs

_____ 23. A specific molecule that stimulates an immune response

_____ 24. The process whereby a drug increases the concentration of certain enzymes that affect the pharmacologic response to another drug

_____ 25. The process whereby a drug blocks enzyme activity and impairs the metabolism of another drug

_____ 26. A change in the action of a drug caused by another drug, a food, or another substance such as alcohol or nicotine

_____ 27. The degree to which a drug or other substance becomes available to the target tissue after administration

_____ 28. The time necessary for the body to eliminate half of the drug in the body at any time; written as $t_{1/2}$

_____ 29. Itching sensation

a. absorption
b. affinity
c. agonist
d. anaphylactic reaction
e. antagonist
f. antigen
g. bioavailability
h. blood-brain barrier
i. ceiling effect
j. dependence
k. distribution
l. elimination
m. first-pass effect
n. half-life
o. induction
p. inhibition
q. interaction
r. lipid
s. loading dose
t. local effect
u. maintenance dose
v. metabolism
w. pharmacokinetics
x. prophylaxis
y. pruritus
z. receptor
aa. solubility
bb. systemic effect
cc. therapeutic range
dd. urticaria

_____ 30. A barrier that prevents many substances from entering the cerebrospinal fluid from the blood; formed by glial cells that envelop the capillaries in the central nervous system, presenting a barrier to many water-soluble compounds though they are permeable to lipid-soluble substances

_____ 31. The extent to which a drug is metabolized by the liver before reaching systemic circulation

_____ 32. A fatty molecule, an important constituent of cell membranes

_____ 33. An action of a drug that is confined to a specific part of the body

_____ 34. Amount of a drug that will bring the blood concentration rapidly to a therapeutic level

_____ 35. Amount of a drug administered at regular intervals to keep the blood concentration at a therapeutic level

_____ 36. A point at which no chemical response occurs with increased dosage

_____ 37. The process by which drugs are chemically converted to other biochemical compounds

_____ 38. The activity of a drug within the body over a period of time; includes absorption, distribution, metabolism, and elimination

_____ 39. The process by which a drug moves from the blood into other body fluids and tissues and ultimately to its sites of action

_____ 40. A drug's ability to dissolve in body fluids

_____ 41. A state in which a person's body has adapted physiologically to a drug and cannot function without it

_____ 42. The process whereby a drug enters the circulatory system

_____ 43. Removal of a drug or its metabolites from the body by excretion

_____ 44. The optimum dosage, providing the best chance for successful therapy

_____ 45. An action of a drug that has a generalized, all-inclusive effect on the body

_____ 46. Drugs that bind to a particular receptor site and trigger the cell's response in a manner similar to the action of the body's own chemical messenger

_____ 47. Hives

_____ 48. Effect of a drug in preventing infection or disease

Dispensing Medications

Understanding Pharmacology and Pharmacokinetics

1. How can a patient achieve relief with sublingual nitroglycerin when the oral route typically has an absorption phase of 15 to 30 minutes?

   _____

   _____

2. What two age groups require special attention when dispensing drugs? Explain your answer.

   _____

   _____

3. If a patient is vomiting and IV antiemetics are not available, what other route of administration could be considered?

   _____

4. What essential items should be checked when reviewing a prescription?

   _____

   _____

5. If a prescriber wrote a prescription on 12-10-18 and the patient brings it to the pharmacy on 12-12-19, can it be filled?

   _____

6. What are the correct drug administration "rights"?

   _____

7. What are the advantages of administering a drug rectally?

   _____

   _____

Name _____ **Date** _____

8. List five drugs that are included in the Beers Criteria that should be avoided in older adults.

   _____

   _____

9. The _____ is the part of a prescription that tells the patient how to take the medication.

10. The information that the federal government requires to be dispensed with certain drugs is known as a(n) _____.

11. The _____ route bypasses the first-pass effect and increases bioavailability of a drug.

12. The _____ route uses skin or mucous membrane absorption as a mode of delivery for medication.

13. What are the advantages of e-prescribing?

   _____

14. Why is it important to check the prescription for the appropriate time for the medication to be administered?

   _____

15. Having too many medications to take can cause a decrease in patient _____.

16. What factors can affect absorption of a drug when it is taken orally? _____

17. Histamine produces symptoms commonly known as the _____.

18. Nizatidine (Axid) is an example of an _____ blocker.

19. A histamine reaction causes _____ constriction.

20. A(n) _____ label contains instructions for the patient, as well as the prescriber's name, the date the prescription was filled, and the drug's name.

Matching–Terms and Definitions

a. allergy
b. Beers Criteria
c. buccal
d. adherence
e. e-prescribing
f. histamine
g. inhalation
h. inscription
i. instillation
j. intradermal
k. intramuscular

l. intrathecal
m. intravenous
n. medication reconciliation
o. ophthalmic
p. oral
q. otic
r. polypharmacy
s. prescription
t. signa
u. subcutaneous
v. sublingual

w. systemic
x. topical
y. three times a day
z. twice a day

_____ 21. The process of obtaining a complete and accurate drug profile for a patient at each transition of care

_____ 22. A state of heightened sensitivity as a result of exposure to a particular substance

_____ 23. Administration of a medication through a vein, thereby avoiding the first-pass effect; abbreviated _IV_

_____ 24. A direction for medication to be dispensed to a patient, written by a physician or a qualified licensed prescriber and filled by a pharmacist; referred to as an order when the medication is requested in a hospital setting

_____ 25. A list of drugs for which monitoring is especially important in older adult patients

_____ 26. Between the cheek and the gums

_____ 27. A patient's compliance to the dose schedule and other particular requirements of the specified regimen

_____ 28. The process that allows a prescriber's computer system to talk to the pharmacy's computer system and the medication order/prescription is transmitted to the pharmacy

_____ 29. A chemical produced by the body that evokes the symptoms of an allergic reaction and is blocked by antihistamines

_____ 30. Injected into the spinal column

_____ 31. Injected into a muscle; abbreviated _IM_

_____ 32. Injected into the skin

_____ 33. Administration of a medication drop by drop

_____ 34. Administration of a medication through the respiratory system

_____ 35. Describes a route of administration in which a medication is applied to the surface of the skin or mucous membranes

_____ 36. Describes a route of administration in which a medication is injected into the tissue just beneath the skin

_____ 37. Describes a route of administration in which a medication is placed under the tongue

_____ 38. Describes a route of administration in which a medication is administered through the eye

_____ 39. Administration of a medication by mouth in either a solid form, as a tablet or capsule, or in a liquid form, as a solution or syrup

_____ 40. The concurrent use of multiple medications

_____ 41. A route of administration in which a medication is instilled in the ear

_____ 42. bid

_____ 43. tid

_____ 44. Part of a prescription that provides directions to be included on the label for the patient to follow in taking the medication

_____ 45. Part of a prescription that identifies the name of the drug, the dose, and the quantities of the ingredients

_____ 46. Pertaining to or affecting the body as a whole

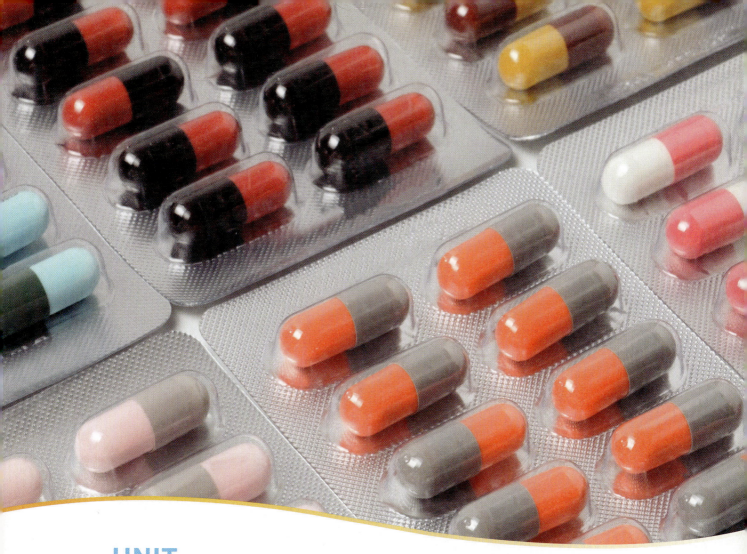

UNIT

2

Major Classes of Pharmaceutical Products I

4

Antibiotics and Antifungals

Reading Drug Labels and Medication Orders

1. A patient brings in the prescription below. The drug label at the right shows the product available in the pharmacy.

> ℞ Amoxil 250 mg/5 mL suspension; take 1 tsp tid × 7 days

a. The concentration requested in the prescription is unavailable. What would the dosing instructions be for the available product? Provide the answer in both teaspoonsfuls and milliliters. (*Note*: 1 tsp = 5 mL. Equivalencies are available in the resources section of Navigator+.)

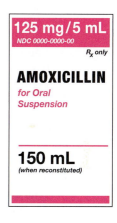

_____

_____

b. Using the drug shown in the label, how many milliliters would you dispense to meet the dosing requirements for the entire treatment period? (Do not assume any wasted medication.)

_____

c. How many milligrams are prescribed for the patient to take in one day?

_____

2. A prescription is written for Augmentin for strep throat. The insurance company refuses to pay for it. When you call the prescriber to change the drug, what do you recommend?

_____

_____

Name _____ Date _____

3. You receive the following prescription:

> ℞ Bactrim DS; 1 tab PO bid × 3d

    a. What directions should be on the dispensed prescription label?

_____

    b. How many tablets will be dispensed for the duration of therapy?

_____

4. You receive an order in your IV room for gentamicin 400 mg. The drug label at the right shows the product available in the pharmacy. How many milliliters would you use to make the dose?

_____

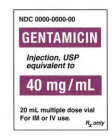

NDC 0000-0000-00

GENTAMICIN

Injection, USP equivalent to

40 mg / mL

20 mL multiple dose vial
For IM or IV use.
     R$_x$ only

5. You receive a prescription that is somewhat difficult to read. The requested drug is either ampicillin or amoxicillin. The drug is dosed three times a day. Which drug do you suspect it is? Why? Who would you verify this information with?

_____

6. Your hospital pharmacy makes a fortified tobramycin eyedrop that is 13.6% in a 10 mL bottle. How many milligrams of the drug are in the bottle of eyedrops?

_____

_____

7. You have an unusual order for intravitreal ceftazidime 2.25 mg/0.1 mL. Your pharmacy has ceftazidime already in solution at 100 mg/mL. Using 1 mL of that ceftazidime, how many milliliters of sodium chloride 0.9% would you have to add to prepare the proper concentration?

_____

_____

8. The following pediatric prescription is received by the pharmacy. The drug label at the right shows the drug to be dispensed.

> ℞ clindamycin 285 mg PO q8 h

100mL   NDC 0000-0000-00

CLINDAMYCIN
Oral Solution

75 mg/5 mL

     R$_x$ only

    a. What are the correct dosing instructions, in milliliters, for the dispensed label?

_____

    b. According to the label, how many doses are in the container?

_____

9. You receive an order for 1,200,000 units of penicillin G for a pediatric patient. The drug label shows the solution available in stock. How many milliliters will provide the dose required?

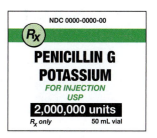

NDC 0000-0000-00

Rx

PENICILLIN G POTASSIUM

FOR INJECTION
USP

2,000,000 units

Rx only   50 mL vial

_____

_____

10. You receive the following prescription:

Rx   Macrobid 100 mg capsules PO bid × 14 days

a. How should the dosing instructions on the dispensed label read?

_____

b. How many 100 mg capsules will be needed for a 14-day supply?

_____

Understanding the Larger Medical Context

11. What is meant by the term *loading dose*?

_____

12. Timmy Thompson is a 13-year-old boy who has severe acne. He is the star right fielder for his Little League team, and he intends to spend most of his summer outside playing baseball. The physician writes the following prescription to treat Timmy's acne:

Rx   minocycline 100 mg PO daily

a. What would you warn Timmy's parents about when they pick up the medication? Other than discontinuing the medication, how could this side effect be managed?

_____

b. How should Timmy change his diet while taking this medication?

_____

13. Mr. Chin calls your pharmacy because he cannot read the instructions for his new Z-Pak prescription. He says, "I have six tablets. Should I take them all at once, or one a day? Should I take this drug on an empty stomach?" What are the instructions Mr. Chin needs to take his Z-Pak?

_____

_____

14. Make a list of the liquid antibiotics that must be stored in the refrigerator (Keep a copy of this list in your pocket for quick reference during your rotations.)

_____

15. Which antibiotic must be mixed in at least 250 mL of fluid and infused slowly to avoid red man syndrome?

    _____

16. Which antibiotic is effective against fungi and protozoa as well as bacteria?

    _____

17. Dr. Patel is a pharmacist who likes to quiz pharmacy technicians about antibiotics. What do you answer when he asks you, "What is the only fourth-generation cephalosporin?"

    _____

18. Clindamycin is the most commonly used lincosamide. What is a caution to clindamycin use?

    _____

Dispensing and Storing Drugs

Where or how should the following medications be stored in the pharmacy?

19. Amoxil suspension

    _____

20. amoxicillin-clavulanate suspension

    _____

21. azithromycin

    _____

22. cefdinir

    _____

23. ampicillin

    _____

24. doxycycline

    _____

25. penicillin

    _____

26. linezolid

    _____

27. reconstituted cefoxitin

    _____

28. clindamycin oral solution

    _____

Putting Safety First

Do the doses match the medications? If not, give a common dose.

29. amoxicillin 2 mg for prophylactic dose for dental procedures

_____

30. Zithromax 1,000 mg

_____

31. amoxicillin tid

_____

32. Fortaz 1-2 g every 8-12 hr

_____

33. Zithromax 1 g to treat chlamydia in women

_____

Understanding Concepts

34. Which antibiotic is also effective against fungi?

_____

35. You receive the following prescription for a 4-year-old patient:

> R℞ clindamycin 150 mg tid for 10 days

Clindamycin is available in 100 mL containers at 75 mg/5 mL. (Remember, all reconstituted antibiotics must be shaken to get the proper dose, because they tend to settle.) What sig will you put on the container? How many containers will you dispense? Where will you tell the parent to store the suspension? What flavor is the suspension?

_____

36. The patient received the following prescription from the dentist:

> R℞ Penicillin 2 g 30 minutes before procedure

When you enter the prescription into the computer, it alerts you that the patient is allergic to penicillin. What do you do?

_____

37. What medication options are available to a dentist who wishes to offer his or her patient a prophylaxis before a procedure?

_____

38. List the antibiotics that must have a medication guide.

   _____

39. List the black box warnings associated with ketoconazole.

   _____

40. Which drug is used for *Clostridium difficile*?

   _____

41. Ciprofloxacin is available in several formulations. You receive a prescription that states:

   ℞   instill 4 gtt AU bid

   Which drug formulation will you choose? What will be the sig on the container?

   _____

42. Your next prescription for ciprofloxacin states the following:

   ℞   instill 1 gtt ou in the a.m. and p.m.

   Which drug formulation will you choose? How will the sig on the container read?

   _____

43. You receive the following prescription for a 25-year-old patient:

   ℞   Bactrim DS BID × 10 days for UTI

   What generic drug will you dispense? What will the sig be? What is UTI? After dispensing the medication, what will you do with the counting tray?

   _____

   _____

   _____

44. The patient, a 9 year old named LaTania, is prescribed Augmentin. Her mother informs you that her child dislikes the orange flavor of the drug. What do you do?

   _____

   _____

Matching–Brand and Generic Drug Names

_____ 45. Adoxa

_____ 46. Amoxil

_____ 47. Augmentin

_____ 48. Bactrim DS

_____ 49. Cipro

_____ 50. Cleocin

_____ 51. Flagyl

_____ 52. Keflex

_____ 53. Omnicef

_____ 54. Z-Pak

a. amoxicillin

b. amoxicillin-clavulanate

c. azithromycin

d. cefdinir

e. cephalexin

f. doxycycline

g. ciprofloxacin

h. clindamycin

i. metronidazole

j. sulfamethoxazole-trimethoprim

Matching–Terms and Definitions

_____ 55. An antibiotic that is effective against multiple organisms

_____ 56. A condition in which bacteria grow in body tissues and cause tissue damage to the host either by their presence or by toxins they produce

_____ 57. A sometimes fatal form of erythema multiforme (an allergic reaction marked by red blotches on the skin)

_____ 58. Low blood pressure

_____ 59. A measurement of acidity or alkalinity

_____ 60. Causing or capable of causing disease or infection

_____ 61. A systemic inflammatory response to infection resulting from blood-borne infections

_____ 62. Treatment begun before a definite diagnosis can be obtained

_____ 63. A chemical substance with the ability to kill or inhibit the growth of bacteria by interfering with bacteria life processes

a. antibiotic

b. broad-spectrum antibiotic

c. empirical treatment

d. hypotension

e. infection

f. pH

g. sepsis

h. Stevens-Johnson syndrome

i. pathogenic

5

Viral Infection Therapy and Acquired Immunity

Reading Drug Labels and Medication Orders

1. You are presented with the following prescription.

> ℞ oseltamivir 75 mg PO BID x 5 days

a. What is the brand name for oseltamivir?

_____

b. You check the pharmacy stock and find you have oseltamivir in 30 mg and 45 mg capsules. How many of each capsule would you dispense for this prescription? Show your calculation.

_____

_____

_____

c. Oseltamivir is also available as an oral suspension with a concentration of 6 mg/mL. If the patient needed a liquid preparation, how many total milliliters would you dispense for the prescription? Show your work.

_____

_____

_____

Name _____ Date _____

2. You are presented with the following prescription, and the drug label shows that the product is available in the pharmacy in 500 mg tablets.

> ℞   Valtrex (valacyclovir) 1 g PO bid × 10 days

a. How many tablets will you dispense? Explain your answer.

_____

_____

_____

b. How will the instructions read on the medication container label?

_____

3. Ms. Roselli brings in the following prescription for her son Joey. Because Joey cannot swallow tablets, she asks you to fill the prescription with a liquid form. You have amantadine syrup 50 mg/5 mL in stock. (*Note*: 1 tsp = 5 mL. Equivalencies are available in the resources section of the Course Navigator.)

> ℞   amantadine 100 mg PO bid × 3 days

a. How many milliliters are in one dose?

_____

b. How many teaspoonsful are in one dose?

_____

c. How will the instructions read on the medication container label?

_____

d. How many milliliters will you dispense?

_____

4. The following medication order is received by the hospital pharmacy for a patient who weighs 184 lb. (*Note*: 1 kg = 2.2 lb. Equivalencies are available in the resources section of the Course Navigator.)

> ℞   acyclovir 10 mg/kg IV q8 h

a. What is the total amount of acyclovir per dose?

_____

b. Using a 50 mg/mL vial, how many milliliters would you use per day?

_____

c. The maximum concentration for acyclovir to be infused is 7 mg/mL. What is the minimum volume to administer this dose? Use the IV solutions available commercially (50 mL, 100 mL, 150 mL, 250 mL, 500 mL, and 1,000 mL).

_____

5. Chapter 3 contains a list of drugs that must be dispensed in the original containers. Which drugs found in this chapter are on that list?

_____

6. You receive the following prescription, and the drug label shows that the product is available:

> ℞ Videx (didanosine) suspension 100 mg PO bid

NDC 0000-0000-00

DIDANOSINE

Pediatric Powder for Oral Solution

R$_x$ only

4 g

a. How would you reconstitute the powder in the container?

_____

_____

b. What volume of didanosine liquid would the patient take per day?

_____

c. Assuming that the dose does not change, how many days will a 200 mL container last?

_____

7. Amantadine, rimantadine, and ranitidine can be easily confused. What is one way they can be distinguished?

_____

8. You receive the following prescription, and the drug label indicates that the drug is available as 450 mg tablets:

> ℞ valganciclovir 900 mg PO bid x 21 days, then 900 mg PO qday

a. How many tablets will be required for a 30-day supply? Show your calculations.

_____

_____

b. What is another dosage form for valganciclovir?

_____

9. You receive the following prescription:

> ℞ saquinavir 600 mg PO tid on an empty stomach

a. What is the brand name of saquinavir?

_____

b. What other drug must be taken with saquinavir?

_____

10. You receive the following prescription.

> ℞   stavudine 30 mg PO BID

a. What is the brand name of this drug?

_____

b. Your pharmacy stocks stavudine in 30 mg capsules. How many capsules would you need to dispense for a 90-day supply?

_____

_____

Understanding the Larger Medical Context

11. Which vaccine may be contraindicated in patients with latex allergy?

_____

_____

12. Which medications are prescribed to patients who have or have been exposed to influenza?

_____

13. Which NNRTI can cause a patient to test positive when taking a cannabinoid (marijuana) test?

_____

14. Which protease inhibitor may cause the patient's skin to turn yellow?

_____

15. Atripla is a combination of which three drugs?

_____

Dispensing and Storing Drugs

16. Which HIV drug must be dispensed with a card for the patient to carry at all times?

_____

17. With which antiviral should you use chemotherapeutic precautions?

_____

18. Which antiviral presented in this chapter is available in both injectable and oral dosage forms?

_____

19. Which anti-influenza agent is available as a powder for inhalation?

_____

20. Which antiherpes agents are prodrugs?

_____

21. Which HIV medication is a prodrug?

_____

22. Which HIV drug is contraindicated in patients currently using allopurinol or ribavirin?

_____

23. Which antiherpes agent should be used with caution in patients with milk sensitivities?

_____

24. Which anti-influenza agent should be used with caution in patients with milk sensitivities?

_____

25. Which drug classes are used to treat HIV?

_____

26. Which vaccines are contraindicated in patients younger than six weeks of age?

_____

27. Which vaccines are contraindicated in patients with yeast hypersensitivity?

_____

28. Which protease inhibitor must be dispensed in the original container?

_____

29. Why have manufacturers of HIV drugs moved to drug combinations?

_____

30. Which drug decreases the effectiveness of stavudine?

_____

Putting Safety First

Does the requested dose match the typical adult medication dose in the following orders? If not, provide the typical adult dosage for each medication.

31. Acyclovir 500 mg PO TID for chronic suppression of genital herpes

_____

32. Valacyclovir 1 g PO BID for chronic suppression of genital herpes

_____

33. Amantadine is packaged in 500 mg doses.

_____

34. Oseltamivir 150 mg PO BID

_____

35. Relenza 2 inhalations bid q12 h for 10 days

_____

Understanding Concepts

36. Why are viral infections generally more difficult to treat compared with bacterial infections?

_____

37. What is the mechanism of action of acyclovir?

_____

38. Which patients are at increased risk of developing complications of influenza?

_____

39. Which brand-name drug is a combination of lopinavir and ritonavir?

_____

40. What is meant by an HIV drug cocktail?

_____

41. What is unique about abacavir that makes it a valuable HIV medication?

_____

42. To which drug class do abacavir and lamivudine belong?

_____

43. What does PEP stand for?

_____

44. Why are HIV medication regimens difficult for patients to adhere to?

_____

45. Which NNRTI decreases the effectiveness of oral contraceptives?

_____

46. Atripla is a combination of which three drug classes? Why does it have a black box warning?

_____

_____

47. What are the two main types of vaccines available?

_____

48. What agency in the United States makes vaccine recommendations? What is its Canadian counterpart?

_____

Matching–Terms and Definitions

_____ 49. One drug given to increase the serum concentration of another drug

_____ 50. vaccines that use pathogens that have been killed with chemicals, heat, or radiation

_____ 51. Tamiflu

_____ 52. the ability of a virus to lie dormant and then, under certain conditions, reproduce and again behave like an infective agent, causing cell damage

_____ 53. Norvir

_____ 54. inflammation of the liver

_____ 55. a virus that can copy its RNA genetic information into the host's DNA

_____ 56. A retrovirus transmitted in body fluids that causes acquired immune deficiency syndrome (AIDS) by attacking T lymphocytes

_____ 57. Having a deficiency in the immune system response

a. boost

b. inactivated vaccines

c. hepatitis

d. human immunodeficiency virus (HIV)

e. immunocompromised

f. retrovirus

g. latency

h. oseltamivir

i. ritonavir

Matching–Antiviral and Antifungal Drugs

Identify whether the drug is an NNRTI, a PI, or a fusion inhibitor (FI).

_____ 58. enfuvirtide (Fuzeon)

_____ 59. atazanavir (Reyataz)

_____ 60. ritonavir (Norvir)

_____ 61. efavirenz (Sustiva)

_____ 62. nevirapine (Viramune)

_____ 63. fosamprenavir (Lexiva)

_____ 64. etravirine (Intelence)

_____ 65. nelfinavir (Viracept)

_____ 66. rilpivirine (Edurant)

_____ 67. delavirdine (Rescriptor)

_____ 68. lopinavir-ritonavir (Kaletra)

_____ 69. darunavir (Prezista)

6

Anesthetics and Narcotics

Reading Drug Labels and Medication Orders

1. In the outpatient pharmacy, you receive the following prescription:

   ℞ Vicodin 5/300 2 tab q4 h prn pain #150

   a. Is this prescription okay to dispense? Explain your answer.

   _____

   b. If the patient takes the prescription as written, what would be the total daily dose of acetaminophen?

   _____

2. What is the fifth vital sign?

   _____

3. What is a PCA pump? Explain the concept.

   _____

   _____

   _____

4. What drug is the standard narcotic analgesic?

   _____

5. What is the result of stimulating the chemoreceptor trigger zone?

   _____

   _____

6. What are the two categories of treatment for migraine headaches?

   _____

Name _____   Date _____

7. How should persistent pain be treated? (Hint: analgesic ladder)

_____

8. Why are the acetaminophen and aspirin components of combination narcotic-nonnarcotic analgesic drugs important?

_____

_____

9. Why are neuromuscular blocking agents important?

_____

10. When is prophylactic treatment indicated for migraines?

_____

11. Which drug is approved for the treatment of hiccups?

_____

Understanding the Larger Medical Context

12. The most common neurotransmitter in the brain is _____, and it is always stimulatory.

13. You work in a children's hospital. Many inhaled anesthetics are kept in stock, but desflurane is not. Why is desflurane unavailable?

_____

_____

14. What is the dose equivalent of Percocet to 10 mg IM morphine?

_____

15. Which class of local anesthetic metabolized by liver enzymes should be avoided in patients with liver insufficiency?

_____

16. Is ketamine (Ketalar) an appropriate anesthetic for a patient with uncontrolled hypertension? Why or why not?

_____

_____

17. Does the autonomic nervous system regulate body systems under voluntary or involuntary control?

_____

18. What are the five components of a classic migraine headache?

_____

_____

19. What drug class is associated with for eletriptan (Relpax)?

_____

20. What dosage forms are commercially available for metoclopramide (Reglan)?

_____

21. Why would you find flumazenil (Romazicon) in an emergency room kit? What are possible side effects of flumazenil?

_____

_____

_____

Dispensing and Storing Drugs

22. Where are schedule II drugs typically kept in the pharmacy, and how are they accessed?

_____

23. Which scheduled drug class must have the original, signed hard copy of the prescription in the pharmacy in some states?

_____

24. Can schedule II drugs be e-prescribed?

_____

25. What form is used when ordering schedule II drugs?

_____

26. Some pharmacies require a count back on some controlled substances. What action is taken in a count back?

_____

_____

Putting Safety First

27. Lidocaine and Duragesic are both available as patches to control pain. Which patch may be cut with scissors to fit a smaller area?

_____

28. What are the prescription limitations of schedule III and schedule IV controlled substances?

_____

29. How many refills are allowed on schedule III and schedule IV prescriptions?

_____

30. How many refills are allowed on schedule II prescriptions?

_____

31. Why are controlled substances so tightly regulated?

_____

Understanding Concepts

32. The _____ _____system transmits information from sensory receptors to the CNS.

33. The only neurotransmitter of the somatic nervous system is _____.

34. The drug derived from fungi and used for migraine treatment is _____.

35. _____ anesthesia is characterized by reversible unconsciousness.

36. The abbreviation for the part of a hospital that provides intensive care is _____.

37. A compulsive disorder that leads to continued use of a drug is _____.

38. CTZ stands for _____.

39. A(n) _____ is a sensation that precedes the onset of a migraine headache.

40. A severe headache may be a _____.

41. A(n) _____ is an electrical signal that travels down the axon of a neuron and ends at the axon terminal.

42. Indicate the controlled-substance schedule for each of the following drugs:

    a. hydromorphone _____

    b. hydrocodone _____

    c. oxycodone _____

    d. morphine _____

    e. diazepam _____

Matching–Brand and Generic Drug Names

_____ 43. acetaminophen-codeine

_____ 44. diazepam

_____ 45. hydrocodone-acetaminophen

_____ 46. lorazepam

_____ 47. metoclopramide

_____ 48. oxycodone-acetaminophen

_____ 49. hydromorphone

_____ 50. sumatriptan

a. Ativan

b. Dilaudid

c. Imitrex

d. Percocet

e. Lortab

f. Reglan

g. Tylenol with Codeine

h. Valium

Matching–Terms and Definitions

_____ 51. addiction

_____ 52. analgesic

_____ 53. analgesic ladder

_____ 54. antagonists

_____ 55. aura

_____ 56. autonomic nervous system

_____ 57. beta-1 receptors

_____ 58. beta-2 receptors

_____ 59. central nervous system

_____ 60. dependence

_____ 61. general anesthesia

_____ 62. local anesthesia

_____ 63. malignant hyperthermia

_____ 64. migraine headache

_____ 65. narcotic analgesic

_____ 66. neurotransmitter

_____ 67. nonsteroidal anti-inflammatory drug

a. A chemical substance that is selectively released from a neuron and stimulates or inhibits activity in the neuron's target cell

b. A compulsive disorder that leads to continued use of a drug despite harm to the user

c. A condition characterized by reversible unconsciousness, analgesia, skeletal muscle relaxation, and amnesia on recovery

d. A drug such as aspirin or ibuprofen that reduces pain and inflammation

e. A drug that alleviates pain

f. A guideline for selecting pain-relieving medications according to the severity of the pain and whether agents lower on the scale have been able to control the pain

g. A physical and emotional reliance on a drug

h. A rare but serious side effect of anesthesia associated with an increase in intracellular calcium and a rapid rise in body temperature

i. A severe throbbing unilateral headache, usually accompanied by nausea, photophobia, phonophobia, and hyperesthesia

j. A subjective sensation or motor phenomenon that precedes and marks the onset of a migraine headache

k. Drugs used to reverse the effects of other drugs, such as in treatment of benzodiazepine or narcotic overdoses

l. Nerve receptors on the heart that control the rate and strength of the heartbeat in response to epinephrine

m. Nerve receptors that control vasodilation and relaxation of the smooth muscle of the airways in response to epinephrine

n. Pain medication containing an opioid

o. The brain and spinal cord

p. The part of the efferent system of the PNS that regulates activities of body structures not under voluntary control

q. The production of transient and reversible loss of sensation in a defined area of the body

7

Psychiatric and Related Drugs

Reading Drug Labels and Medication Orders

1. You receive a prescription that indicates the patient is to take "500 mg qam for 10 days." The medication is available in 250 mg tablets.

   a. How many tablets will the patient take in a day?

   _____

   b. How many tablets will be dispensed?

   _____

2. You receive the following prescription. Celexa comes in a 240 mL container, in an oral solution of 10 mg/5 mL.

   ℞   Celexa oral solution 30 mg PO a day

   a. How much liquid will be in each dose?

   _____

   b. How long will the container last the patient?

   _____

Name _____   Date _____

Understanding the Larger Medical Context

3. List three side effects of tricyclic antidepressants.

   _____

4. What side effect of some antipsychotic medications causes involuntary movements and may be irreversible?

   _____

5. Why is clozapine not more commonly used?

   _____

   _____

   _____

6. List three side effects of atypical antipsychotics.

   _____

   _____

   _____

7. Which antidepressant works only on dopamine receptors?

   _____

8. MAOIs have many side effects and are used less frequently now to treat psychotic disorders. What other use do these drugs have?

   _____

9. Which atypical antipsychotics are available as injectables? What is the advantage of using injectable atypical antipsychotics?

   _____

Dispensing and Storing Drugs

10. Which OTC classes of medications are used for insomnia?

    _____

11. With which drug will patients commonly self-medicate their anxiety?

    _____

12. What are the effects of tardive dyskinesia?

    _____

13. Which drugs are stored near and could easily be confused with Celebrex?

    _____

14. Which drug is often confused with Pepcid because it has a similar-sounding name and is available in the same strength?

_____

15. What type of drugs in this chapter must have a medication guide?

_____

16. Which tricyclic antidepressant is used in the liquid form by dentists to treat "burning mouth" syndrome?

_____

_____

Fill in the blanks with the controlled-substance schedule for each of the following drugs.

_____ 17. armodafinil (Nuvigil)

_____ 18. zolpidem (Ambien)

_____ 19. benzodiazepines

_____ 20. modafinil (Provigil)

_____ 21. eszopiclone (Lunesta)

_____ 22. ramelteon (Rozerem)

Putting Safety First

23. Why should trazodone be avoided in young males?

_____

24. You receive the following prescription:

> ℞   Xanax 1 mg tid #90 refills 11

Can you fill the prescription as written? Why or why not?

_____

25. A prescription for a schedule II drug is presented to you. It has two refills on it and no DEA number. Can this prescription be filled? Why or why not?

_____

Understanding Concepts

26. Compare and contrast depression and bipolar disorder.

   _____

27. What is serotonin?

   _____

28. Why are atypical antipsychotics used more frequently than typical or first-generation antipsychotics?

   _____

29. Describe how disulfiram works in patients with alcohol dependence.

   _____

30. List four symptoms of alcohol dependence.

   _____

   _____

   _____

   _____

31. Which drug class may be used for bed-wetting problems in children?

   _____

32. Which antidepressant drug is approved as an aid to smoking cessation?

   _____

33. Which hypnotic is not a controlled substance?

   _____

34. What is the brand name of haloperidol?

   _____

35. Which hypnotic drug is approved to treat sleep-onset insomnia?

   _____

36. Which drug is prescribed to treat bipolar disorder and is also the name of a metal?

   _____

37. What is the generic name for Seroquel?

   _____

38. What is the brand name for temazepam?

   _____

39. What is the generic name for Prozac?

_____

40. Which chronic psychotic disorder is marked by delusions, bizarre behavior, withdrawal, and abnormalities in perception and content of thought?

_____

41. What is the advantage of prescribing bupropion over other antidepressants for older adult males?

_____

42. _____ _____ is an intense, overwhelming, and uncontrollable anxiety.

43. _____ dyskinesia is characterized by involuntary movements of the mouth, lips, and tongue.

44. _____ is a state of uneasiness characterized by apprehension and worry about possible events.

45. _____ uses an osmotic controlled-release oral delivery system.

46. _____ is a pattern of alcohol use that involves problems controlling drinking, preoccupation with alcohol, use of alcohol even when it causes problems, drinking more to get the same effect, or having withdrawal symptoms with rapidly decreasing or stopping drinking.

47. _____ disorder is a condition in which patients swing between major depression and agitation.

48. Difficulty falling and/or staying asleep is referred to as _____.

49. _____ was originally referred to as "shell shock."

50. _____ is a form of depression that occurs in fall and winter.

Matching–Brand and Generic Drug Names

_____ 51. alprazolam

_____ 52. bupropion

_____ 53. buspirone

_____ 54. citalopram

_____ 55. diazepam

_____ 56. escitalopram

_____ 57. eszopiclone

_____ 58. fluoxetine

_____ 59. lorazepam

_____ 60. olanzapine

_____ 61. quetiapine

_____ 62. risperidone

_____ 63. temazepam

_____ 64. trazodone

_____ 65. venlafaxine

_____ 66. zolpidem

a. Ambien

b. Ativan

c. BuSpar

d. Celexa

e. Desyrel

f. Effexor

g. Lexapro

h. Lunesta

i. Prozac

j. Restoril

k. Risperdal

l. Seroquel

m. Valium

n. Wellbutrin

o. Xanax

p. Zyprexa

Matching–Terms and Definitions

_____ 67. A condition in which a patient presents with mood swings that alternate between periods of major depression and periods of mild to severe chronic agitation

_____ 68. A state of uneasiness characterized by apprehension and worry about possible events

_____ 69. A possibly fatal condition caused by combining antidepressants that increase serotonin levels with other medications that also stimulate serotonin receptors

_____ 70. A class of antidepressant drugs, developed earlier than the SSRIs and SNRIs, that also prevent neuron reuptake of norepinephrine and/or serotonin

_____ 71. An antidepressant drug that inhibits the activity of the enzymes that break down catecholamines (such as norepinephrine) and serotonin

_____ 72. Empty shell of an OROS tablet, excreted in the stool after the drug has dissolved

_____ 73. A drug that induces sleep

_____ 74. An antidepressant drug that blocks the reuptake of serotonin with little effect on norepinephrine and fewer side effects than other antidepressant drugs

_____ 75. A drug delivery system that allows the drug to dissolve through pores in the tablet shell; the empty shell, is passed in the stool

a. anxiety

b. bipolar disorder

c. ghost tablet

d. hypnotic

e. monoamine oxidase inhibitor (MAOIs)

f. osmotic-controlled release oral delivery system (OROS)

g. selective serotonin reuptake inhibitor (SSRI)

h. serotonin syndrome

i. tricyclic antidepressant (TCA)

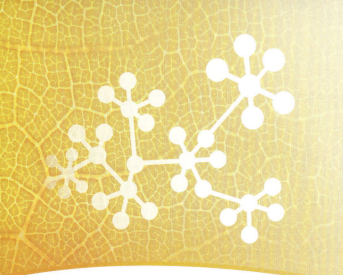

8

Drugs for Central Nervous System Disorders

Reading Drug Labels and Medication Orders

1. You receive the following prescription. What is the problem with the prescription as written?

   ℞ methylphenidate 30 mg PO 1 bid #60 refill × 11

   _____

2. You receive the following prescription, and the drug label shown is the product available in the pharmacy. How many tablets will you dispense? Show your calculations.

   ℞ Dilantin 50 mg bid × 2 days, then 50 mg qid × 8 days

   _____
   _____
   _____

   NDC 0000-0000-00

   ## Phenytoin

   ### 50 mg

   Caution: Federal law prohibits dispensing without prescription

   100 tablets

Name _____ Date _____

3. You receive the following order for a patient who weighs 88 kg. The pharmacy has azathioprine in 100 mg vials.

R̶ Imuran IV 1.75 mg/kg/day

a. What is the daily dose? Show your calculations.

_____

b. How much product would be used in a six-day supply? Show your calculations.

_____

Understanding the Larger Medical Context

4. What are the different types of generalized seizures?

_____

_____

5. What region of the brain loses dopaminergic neurons, which results in the onset of Parkinson's disease?

_____

6. What is the benefit of using the combination drug levodopa-carbidopa to treat Parkinson's disease rather than levodopa on its own?

_____

_____

_____

_____

7. What is the most common reason for drug therapy failure in patients who have epilepsy?

_____

_____

8. What are three drugs to treat status epilepticus?

_____

_____

_____

9. What are signs and symptoms of myasthenia gravis?

_____

_____

_____

_____

10. Which two drugs are approved to treat fibromyalgia?

_____

Dispensing and Storing Drugs

Where or how should the following medications be stored in the pharmacy?

11. glatiramer acetate (Copaxone)

_____

12. interferon beta-1a (Avonex)

_____

13. What auxiliary label would you affix to the interferon beta-1a (Avonex) container?

_____

14. Focalin XR is the extended-release form of which generic drug?

_____

15. List the drugs in this chapter that require a medication guide. Remember to list them individually, not as a class.

_____

Name the controlled-substance schedule for each of the following drugs.

_____ 16. dexmethylphenidate (Focalin)

_____ 17. dextroamphetamine-amphetamine (Adderall)

_____ 18. lisdexamfetamine (Vyvanse)

_____ 19. lacosamide (Vimpat)

_____ 20. methylphenidate (Concerta)

_____ 21. phenobarbital (Luminal)

_____ 22. pregabalin (Lyrica)

Putting Safety First

Does the requested dose match the typical medication dose in the following orders? If not, provide the typical dosage for each medication.

23. Zarontin bid to achieve therapeutic plasma concentrations

   _____

24. Keppra should be given in doses greater than 3,000 mg to be effective.

   _____

   _____

25. Zelapar daily dose should not exceed 10 mg.

   _____

26. Concerta bid

   _____

27. Interferon beta-1a administered every other day

   _____

Understanding Concepts

28. Which drug is formulated using an osmotic-release oral delivery system?

   _____

29. _____ acid is an anticonvulsant.

30. _____ is a combination of levodopa, carbidopa, and entacapone.

31. _____ is the generic name for Symmetrel.

32. A _____ seizure is a serious form of seizure.

33. _____ gravis is a disorder of the interface between nerves and muscles, resulting in the muscles being unresponsive to nerve signals to move them.

34. _____ is an autoimmune disease that affects the myelin sheaths around nerves.

35. _____ is a neurologic disorder involving sudden and recurring seizures.

36. The _____ oblongata is a part of the brain.

37. _____ leg syndrome causes pain or unpleasant sensations in the legs, especially after retiring to bed.

38. _____ is characterized by long-term pain across the entire body, as well as tenderness in the joints, muscles, and tendons.

39. _____ epilepticus is a serious disorder involving continuous tonic-clonic convulsions.

40. A _____ seizure is localized in a specific area of the brain and almost always results from injury to the cerebral cortex.

41. _____ is a neurological disorder that involves sudden and recurring seizures.

42. Which nonstimulant drug is used to treat ADHD? _____

43. List the drugs used to treat Parkinson's disease that are MAOIs.

   _____

44. Which drug is used to treat Parkinson's disease and influenza?

   _____

45. _____ is the most commonly used drug in the treatment of Parkinson's disease.

46. _____ is structurally similar to gabapentin.

Matching–Brand and Generic Drug Names

_____ 47. atomoxetine

_____ 48. primidone

_____ 49. dextroamphetamine-amphetamine

_____ 50. divalproex

_____ 51. gabapentin

_____ 52. lamotrigine

_____ 53. valproic acid

a. Adderall

b. Depakene

c. Depakote

d. Mysoline

e. Lamictal

f. Neurontin

g. Strattera

Matching–Terms and Definitions

_____ 54. adjunct

_____ 55. Alzheimer's disease

_____ 56. amyotrophic lateral sclerosis

_____ 57. anticonvulsant

_____ 58. attention-deficit hyperactivity disorder (ADHD)

_____ 59. dysphagia

_____ 60. isomer

_____ 61. on-off phenomenon

_____ 62. Parkinson's disease

_____ 63. restless leg syndrome

_____ 64. seizure

_____ 65. status epilepticus

_____ 66. GABA

a. A degenerative disorder of the brain that leads to progressive dementia and changes in personality and behavior

b. A degenerative disease of the motor nerves; also called _Lou Gehrig's disease_

c. A drug used to control seizures

d. A drug used with another drug

e. A neurologic disorder characterized by akinesia, resting tremor, and muscle rigidity

f. A neurologic disorder characterized by hyperactivity, impulsivity, and distractibility

g. A neurotransmitter capable of inhibiting neuron firing

h. Difficulty swallowing

i. An overpowering urge to move the legs, especially at rest

j. A serious disorder involving tonic-clonic convulsions that last at least 30 minutes

k. Involuntary contraction or series of contractions of the voluntary muscles

l. One of two or more compounds that contain the same number and type of atoms but have different molecular structures

m. A wide fluctuation between abnormally increased and abnormally diminished motor function; present in many patients who have Parkinson's disease after about five years of levodopa therapy

9

Respiratory Drugs

Reading Drug Labels and Medication Orders

1. Mr. Gaines brings in a prescription for the following cough syrup:

   ℞ Robitussin A-C 1 tsp PO q4-6 h prn persistent cough

   a. How would you express the directions on the label?

   _____

   _____

   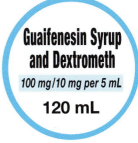

   Guaifenesin Syrup and Dextrometh
   100 mg/10 mg per 5 mL
   120 mL

   b. What auxiliary labels would you add to this prescription bottle? Explain.

   _____

   _____

2. Ms. Marcos presents the following prescription to the pharmacy:

   ℞ Nicotine lozenge PO q4 h prn cravings

   If Ms. Marcos uses the maximum number of lozenges every day, how many would she need for a month? Show your calculations.

   _____

   _____

Name _____ Date _____

3. You receive the following order in the pharmacy:

Ŗ   Singulair 10 mg chew one tab PO daily

a. Which dosage forms for Singulair are available for this order?

_____

b. How many tablets would you supply for one month? Show your calculations.

_____

4. You receive the following prescription in the pharmacy:

Ŗ   cetirizine oral solution 2.5 mg PO daily for 30 days

You check your pharmacy's stock and see that you have two options: 5 mg/5 mL and 1 mg/1 mL.

a. If you dispense from the 5 mg/5 mL bottle, how much would you dispense and what would be the dose? Show your calculations.

_____

b. If you dispense from the 1 mg/mL bottle, how much would you dispense and what would be the dose? Show your calculations.

_____

5. You receive the following prescription:

Ŗ   rifampin 300 mg PO daily

How many 150 mg capsules would the patient require for a three-month supply? Show your calculations.

_____

6. You receive the following order:

Ŗ   Zyban 150 mg PO qhs daily for three days, then 150 mg PO BID x 7 weeks.

a. Based on the prescription, which generic product would you dispense?

_____

b. What are all the dosage forms available for bupropion?

_____

7. You receive the following prescription:

> R_x Claritin 10 mg daily

What dosage form would be most appropriate for the nasogastric route? For the nasogastric route, a plastic tube is inserted through the nose, down the back of the throat, through the esophagus, and into the stomach.

_____

Understanding the Larger Medical Context

8. You receive the following prescription. Which brand name product would you expect to dispense? Explain your answer.

> R_x fluticasone 50 mcg, 1 spray daily in each nostril

_____

_____

9. Mr. Usher takes the following regimen for his asthma:

> R_x Advair 250/50 1 puff bid

What should Mr. Usher do after taking his dose of Advair?

_____

_____

10. When using inhalers, what is the main difference between the HFA MDI inhaler compared to the dry-powder MDI inhaler?

_____

_____

11. List the benefits of not smoking.

_____

_____

_____

Dispensing and Storing Drugs

12. Identify a consideration when storing Spiriva Handihaler capsules.

    _____

13. What is an alternative tiotropium product for patient that has difficulty using the HandiHaler device?

    _____

14. You receive the following prescription:

    > ℞ Duoneb 0.5mg/2.5mg per nebulizer every 4 hours dispense 1 month's supply

    How many mLs will be charged to the insurance company? _____
    (Duoneb comes 0.5mg/2.5mg/3 mL.)

15. Mr. Mkembe brings you this prescription:

    > ℞ Ipatropium 0.02% (500 micrograms/2.5mL) use 500 micrograms in nebulizer four times daily. Dispense one month's supply.

    How many mLs will be billed to the insurance company? _____

16. Which device is dispensed with a metered dose inhaler to help get the drug into the lungs?

    _____

17. Which medications used for tuberculosis should receive an auxiliary label that reads "This drug interferes with the effectiveness of oral contraceptives"?

    _____

Putting Safety First

18. Johnnie Sparza, a four-year-old patient, is using his nebulizer correctly, but he constantly gets bronchial infections. Casually, you ask his mother how often she cleans the nebulizer. She replies, "Oh, every now and then."

    a. What might be the source of Johnnie's infections?

    _____

    b. Explain to Johnnie's mother how often she should clean the nebulizer.

    _____

19. Which drug is made from human plasma and therefore carries the risk of transmitting infections?

    _____

Understanding Concepts

20. _____ is a reversible lung disease.

21. _____ is the addictive component of tobacco.

22. _____ is an agent that destroys mucus.

23. _____ is the measurement used to assess the severity of asthma.

24. _____ is a device used with inhaled medicines.

25. MDI stands for _____.

26. _____ is the drug used in most rescue inhalers.

27. Dulera contains which two drugs? _____

28. _____ work by inhibiting acetylcholine.

29. Which systemic antihistamine has a bitter taste?

_____

Matching–Brand and Generic Drug Names

_____ 30. Advair Diskus

_____ 31. Allegra

_____ 32. Clarinex

_____ 33. Mucinex

_____ 34. Mucinex D

_____ 35. Nasonex

_____ 36. Robitussin A-C

_____ 37. Singulair

_____ 38. Tussionex

_____ 39. Zyrtec

a. cetirizine

b. desloratadine

c. guaifenesin-codeine

d. guaifenesin-pseudoephedrine

e. fluticasone-salmeterol

f. fexofenadine

g. guaifenesin

h. mometasone

i. montelukast

j. hydrocodone-chlorpheniramine

Matching–Terms and Definitions

_____ 40. antihistamines

_____ 41. asthma

_____ 42. antitussives

_____ 43. bronchitis

_____ 44. corticosteroid

_____ 45. cough suppressant

_____ 46. cystic fibrosis

_____ 47. decongestant

_____ 48. expectorant

_____ 49. guaifenesin

_____ 50. metered dose inhaler (MDI)

_____ 51. mucolytic

_____ 52. nebulizer

_____ 53. pseudoephedrine

_____ 54. RDS

_____ 55. rhinitis medicamentosa

_____ 56. spacer

_____ 57. varenicline

_____ 58. xanthine derivative

a. A condition of decreased response that results when nasal decongestants are used over prolonged periods

b. A condition in which the inner lining of the bronchial airways becomes inflamed, causing the expiration of air from the lungs to be obstructed

c. A device that delivers a specific amount of medication (as for asthma) in a fine enough spray to reach the innermost parts of the lungs using a puff of compressed gas

d. A device used in the administration of inhaled medications, using air flowing past a liquid to create a mist

e. A device used with a metered dose inhaler (MDI) to decrease the amount of spray deposited on the back of the throat and swallowed

f. A drug that causes relaxation of the airway smooth muscle, thus causing airway dilation and better air movement

g. A drug that chemically resembles substances produced by the adrenal gland and acts as an anti-inflammatory agent to suppress the immune response by stimulating adenylate cyclase

h. A reversible lung disease with intermittent attacks in which inspiration is obstructed; provoked by airborne allergens

i. An agent that causes the mucous membranes to shrink, thereby allowing the sinus cavities to drain

j. An agent that decreases the thickness and stickiness of mucus, enabling the patient to rid the lungs and airway of mucus when coughing

k. An agent that destroys or dissolves mucus

l. Common term for drugs that block the H_1 receptors

m. Drugs that block or suppress the act of coughing

n. CF

o. dextromethorphan

p. Mucinex

q. stop smoking drug that causes strange dreams

r. Sudafed

s. Respiratory Distress Syndrome

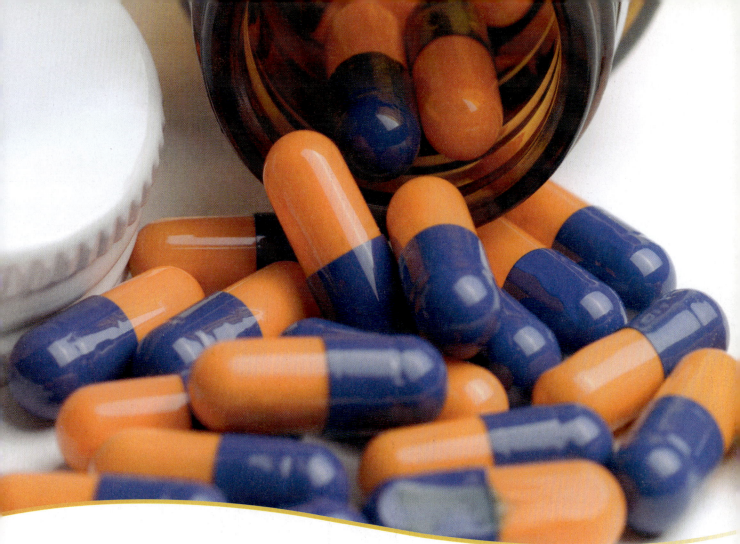

UNIT

3 Major Classes of Pharmaceutical Products II

10

Drugs for Gastrointestinal and Related Diseases

Reading Drug Labels and Medication Orders

1. A patient comes into your pharmacy with the following prescription. If the patient took this medication as frequently as the prescription allows, how long would it take for a pint-sized bottle to run out? Show your calculations.

R̥ Maalox 1 tbsp PO tid prn heartburn

_____

_____

2. Mr. Griffiths has been diagnosed with recurrent gallstones. He is currently using Actigall at prophylaxis doses. The physician has written the following prescription. Based on the smallest available capsule size for this medication, how many capsules will Mr. Griffiths receive in a month?

R̥ Actigall 300 mg PO bid

_____

3. Mrs. Sim has been given a prescription for Enulose, and the following drug label shows the product available in the pharmacy.

R̥ lactulose 2 tbsp PO q6 h prn constipation

Name _____ Date _____

a. How many grams of lactulose will Mrs. Sim get in a dose? Explain.

_____

_____

b. How many doses can Mrs. Sim get from a bottle of lactulose, assuming no waste? Show your calculations.

_____

c. How many days of treatment will a bottle last if Mrs. Sim takes the maximum dosage per day? Show your calculations.

_____

_____

16 Fl Oz (473 mL)

NDC 0000-0000-00

Lactulose Syrup USP

10 g/15 mL ▬▬▬

FOR ORAL OR RECTAL ADMINISTRATION

Each 15 mL of syrup contains 10 g lactulose

Caution: Federal law prohibits dispensing without prescription

4. Mr. Nasser is on mesalamine 800 mg PO tid.

   a. List the brand name products available for mesalamine.

   _____

   b. What will be the directions on the medication label?

   _____

5. Mr. Ngo has been instructed to take Pepto-Bismol for his traveler's diarrhea. What is the generic name for Pepto-Bismol?

   _____

6. Mrs. Anderson, a patient with hepatitis C, brings the following prescription to your pharmacy:

   ℞ Copegus 600 mg PO bid

   a. If the tablets are 200 mg, how many tablets will she receive in one day?

   _____

7. Mr. Doole requires ranitidine in his total parenteral nutrition (TPN) for stress ulcer prophylaxis. The recommended dose is 150 mg/day. How many milliliters of Zantac for injection would Mr. Doole get in each TPN?

   _____

NDC 0000-0000-00

ranitidine hydrochloride Injection

25 mg/mL*

40-mL Pharmacy Bulk Package — Not for Direct Infusion

Sterile   ℞ only

Contents should be used as soon as possible following initial closure puncture. Discard any unused portion within 24 hours of first entry.

* Each 1 mL of aqueous solution contains ranitidine 25 mg (as the hydrochloride); phenol 5 mg as preservative; monobasic potassium phosphate and dibasic sodium phosphate as buffers.

See package insert for Dosage and Administration and directions for use of Pharmacy Bulk Package.

Store between 4° and 25°C (39° and 77°F); excursions permitted to 30°C (86°F). Protect from light. Store vial in carton until time of use.

Understanding the Larger Medical Context

8. Mrs. Copeland comes to the pharmacy and tells you she was diagnosed with an ulcer. She says her prescriber thinks her ulcer may be from using aspirin and ibuprofen. How do these drugs contribute to ulcers?

   _____

   _____

9. To increase the chances for successful treatment of hepatitis C, which medication must be used with Copegus? Why?

   _____

10. Which medication can treat both diarrhea and constipation?

   _____

11. What non-medication measures can be taken to prevent and treat constipation?

   _____

12. Which class of antiemetics is used for treatment of emesis in chemotherapy?

   _____

13. Give two examples of medications from the above class (question 12).

   _____

14. Which types of hepatitis have vaccines for prevention?

   _____

Dispensing and Storing Drugs

15. The pharmacist is pregnant. An order comes down for Cytotec. Should she fill the script? Why or why not?

   _____

16. Which antimotility drugs are controlled?

   _____

17. Which antimotility medication is OTC?

   _____

18. The technician enters a prescription for sulfasalazine for Mr. Yamaguchi. What type of drug allergy or hypersensitivity would contraindicate sulfasalazine use?

   _____

19. Which hepatitis drugs require a medication guide?

   _____

20. The patient is taking a trip abroad and brings in a prescription of for nitazoxanide. The patient has type 2 diabetes and uses metformin. What should the patient be warned about?

_____

21. Why should bulk-forming laxatives be taken with at least eight ounces of water?

_____

22. Which proton pump inhibitors are stored in the OTC area of the store?

_____

Do the doses match the medications? If not, give a common dose.

23. Carafate is dosed every eight hours.

_____

24. Sulfasalazine 2 grams BID ulcerative colitis

_____

25. Lomotil combination of 0.25 mg diphenoxylate and 0.25 mg atropine

_____

26. Lubiprostone 24 mg BID.

_____

27. Methylnaltrexone 12 mcg once daily.

_____

Understanding Concepts

28. _____ is a proton pump inhibitor that has an IV form.

29. _____ is a laxative as well as an antacid.

30. _____ is a bowel evacuant that is OTC and available in powder form.

31. A _____ is a combination of bismuth subcitrate, metronidazole, and tetracycline.

32. _____ forms a protective coat or shield over the ulcer and is dosed every six hours.

33. _____ is a food that can be used to treat nausea.

34. List the serotonin receptor antagonists designed to treat nausea induced by chemotherapy: _____

35. _____ is the brand name of sodium phosphate used as a bowel evacuant.

36. _____ is a proton pump inhibitor that comes in capsule form, and can be opened and mixed with apple sauce for those patients who have difficulty swallowing.

37. _____ is an immunosuppressant used in the treatment of Crohn's disease.

38. _____ massage is a complementary and alternative therapy for nausea.

39. A duodenal _____ is a peptic lesion.

40. _____ is a drug used for travelers diarrhea that does not carry the concern of bacterials resistance.

41. _____ is a combination of calcium carbonate and simethicone.

42. _____ is a schedule IV drug used to treat diarrhea.

43. Most antacids are found in the _____ aisle of the pharmacy.

44. _____ are drugs used in patients with ulcerative colitis and Crohn's disease for their anti-inflammatory and immunosuppressive qualities.

45. _____ are used for induction and maintenance of remission in patients with Crohn's disease and ulcerative colitis.

46. _____ is the notation used for immune globulin that is administered IV.

47. _____ is the abbreviation of a condition characterized by a backflow of stomach acid.

Matching–Brand and Generic Drug Names

_____ 48. famotidine

_____ 49. omeprazole

_____ 50. cimetidine

_____ 51. sucralfate

_____ 52. ursodiol

_____ 53. metoclopramide

_____ 54. nitazoxanide

_____ 55. bisacodyl

_____ 56. lactulose

_____ 57. docusate

_____ 58. ledipasvir/sofosbuvir

a. Prilosec

b. Pepcid

c. Carafate

d. Tagamet

e. Harvoni

f. Colace

g. Reglan

h. Actigall

i. Alinia

j. Enulose

k. Dulcolax

Matching–Terms and Definitions

_____ 59. antiemetic

_____ 60. chemoreceptor trigger zone (CTZ)

_____ 61. gastroesophageal reflux disease (GERD)

_____ 62. histamine H_2 receptor antagonist

_____ 63. hepatitis

_____ 64. IVIG

_____ 65. irritable bowel syndrome (IBS)

_____ 66. osmotic laxative

_____ 67. phenothiazine

_____ 68. proton pump inhibitor

_____ 69. reflux

_____ 70. saline laxative

_____ 71. surfactant laxative

_____ 72. traveler's diarrhea

_____ 73. vertigo

a. A disease of the liver that causes inflammation, can be acute or chronic, and has several forms A through G

b. A drug, related to the typical antipsychotics, that controls vomiting by inhibiting the CTZ

c. A drug that blocks gastric acid secretion by inhibiting the enzyme that pumps hydrogen ions into the stomach

d. A drug that controls nausea and vomiting

e. A GI disease characterized by radiating burning or pain in the chest and an acid taste, caused by backflow of acidic stomach contents across an incompetent lower esophageal sphincter; also referred to as heartburn

f. A functional disorder in which the lower GI tract does not have appropriate tone or spasticity to regulate bowel activity.

g. A stool softener that has a detergent activity that facilitates mixing of fat and water, making the stool soft and mushy

h. An agent that blocks acid and pepsin secretion in response to histamine, gastrin, foods, distention, caffeine, or cholinergic stimulation; used to treat GERD and *H. pylori*

i. An area below the floor of the fourth ventricle of the brain that can trigger nausea and vomiting when certain signals are received

j. An inorganic salt that attracts water into the hollow portion (lumen) of the colon, increasing intraluminal pressure to cause evacuation

k. An organic substance that draws water into the colon and thereby stimulates evacuation

l. Backflow; specifically in GERD, the backflow of acidic stomach contents across an incompetent lower esophageal sphincter

m. Diarrhea caused by ingesting contaminated food or water; so called because it is often contracted by travelers in countries where the water supply is contaminated

n. The notation for immune globulin that is given intravenously

o. The sensation of the room spinning when one gets up or changes positions; can be treated with anticholinergic agents

11

Renal System Drugs

Reading Drug Labels and Medication Orders

1. You receive the following prescription, and the product available in the pharmacy is 5 mg/mL of oral liquid in a 473 mL container:

    ℞   Ditropan Liquid 7 mL bid

    a. How much do you need to dispense for a 30-day supply?

    _____

    b. If you dispensed the entire container, how long would it last the patient?

    _____

2. You receive the following prescription for a product available in the pharmacy:

    ℞   Hiprex 1,000 mg PO BID

    a. What is this prescription for?

    _____

    b. What product should be avoided while taking this drug?

    _____

Name _____   Date _____

3. You receive the following prescription, and the product available in the pharmacy is available as 10 mg/mL in a 120 mL container:

R℞   furosemide liquid 40 mg PO daily

How long will this container last the patient?

_____

4. You receive the following prescription:

R℞   torsemide 20 mg IV every day

The pharmacy has a 2 mL and a 5 mL size of 10 mg/mL. Which of the two products do you choose to fill the prescription? Why?

_____

_____

Understanding the Larger Medical Context

5. Which type of bacteria causes most urinary tract infections?

_____

6. What are side effects of potassium-sparing diuretics?

_____

7. What are the stages of chronic kidney disease?

_____

_____

_____

_____

8. By which three processes do the kidneys produce urine?

_____

_____

_____

9. What is anemia? What role can erythropoietin play in anemia?

_____

_____

_____

Dispensing and Storing Drugs

10. The prescriber wants a carbonic anhydrase inhibitor IV diuretic. Which one will the pharmacy technician prepare?

   _____

11. Which diluent must be used with the IV form of CellCept?

   _____

Indicate which drugs have black box warnings (BBW), medication guides (MG), both (B), or neither (N).

12. Aranesp _____

13. ciprofloxacin _____

14. hydrochlorothiazide _____

15. Oxytrol _____

16. nitrofurantoin _____

17. Uroxatral _____

18. doxazosin _____

19. phenazopyridine _____

20. Epogen _____

21. CellCept _____

22. iron dextran _____

23. Nephrocaps is a brand of vitamins specially formulated for dialysis patients. What does Nephrocaps contain?

   _____

24. What are the two main types of dialysis?

   _____

25. Which drug is a long-acting erythropoietin-stimulating agent?

   _____

26. Which drug used to treat a UTI changes the urine brown or dark yellow?

   _____

27. Which drug has a local anesthetic effect in the urinary tract?

   _____

28. Which alpha blocker is more selective: Flomax (tamsulosin) or Hytrin (terazosin)?

   _____

29. Which drugs are agents for urinary incontinence that decrease urinary frequency?

   _____

30. Where in the kidney does each of the following types of medication work?

   thiazide diuretics
   loop diuretics
   carbonic anhydrase inhibitors
   potassium-sparing diuretics

   a. distal tubule   _____
   b. glomerulus   _____
   c. ascending loop of Henle _____
   d. proximal tubule   _____

Putting Safety First

31. Why is it important to check the laboratory results of patients taking furosemide to see if their potassium levels are appropriate?

      _____

32. List three drug classes that should be avoided in BPH patients.

      _____

33. HCTZ is an abbreviation for what drug?

      _____

34. What is the purpose of adding triamterene to hydrochlorothiazide?

      _____

35. Name two brand names for the combination drug triamterene-hydrochlorothiazide.

      _____

36. _____ is a class of drugs is used to decrease high blood pressure and treat BPH.

37. _____ is a potassium-sparing diuretic that is 100 times more specific in its affinity for aldosterone than spironolactone.

38. _____ is a urinary analgesic that colors the urine orange and stains anything it contacts.

39. _____ is a complementary and alternative product used to prevent UTIs.

40. _____ is also known as prostate gland enlargement.

41. _____ is the frequent need to urinate at night.

42. _____ is the working unit of the kidney.

43. _____ is the removal of substances from the blood during urine formation.

Matching–Brand and Generic Drug Names

_____ 44. Flomax

_____ 45. Microzide

_____ 46. Hyzaar

_____ 47. Lasix

_____ 48. Lozol

_____ 49. Maxzide

_____ 50. Tenoretic

_____ 51. Zestoretic

_____ 52. Ziac

a. indapamide

b. atenolol-chlorthalidone

c. bisoprolol-hydrochlorothiazide

d. furosemide

e. hydrochlorothiazide

f. lisinopril-hydrochlorothiazide

g. losartan-hydrochlorothiazide

h. triamterene-hydrochlorothiazide

i. tamsulosin

Matching–Terms and Definitions

_____ 53. carbonic anhydrase inhibitor

_____ 54. diuretic

_____ 55. hemodialysis

_____ 56. loop diuretic

_____ 57. nocturia

_____ 58. glomerular filtration rate

_____ 59. potassium-sparing diuretic

_____ 60. reabsorption

_____ 61. thiazide diuretic

_____ 62. urinary tract infection (UTI)

a. A diuretic that acts in the proximal tubule to increase urine volume and change the pH from acidic to alkaline

b. A drug that blocks a pump that removes sodium and chloride together from the distal tubule

c. A value used to determine kidney health; an estimate of how much blood passes through glomeruli each minute

d. A drug that inhibits the reabsorption of sodium and chloride in the loop of Henle, thereby causing an increased urinary output

e. A drug that promotes excretion of water and sodium but inhibits the exchange of sodium for potassium

f. A substance that rids the body of excess fluid and electrolytes by increasing the urine output

g. An infection caused by bacteria, usually _E. coli,_ that enter via the urethra and progress up the urinary tract; characterized by the presence of bacteria in the urine with localized symptoms

h. The process by which substances are pulled back into the blood after waste products have been removed during the formation of urine

i. The process of diverting blood flow through a machine that mechanically filters blood and returns blood to the body

j. Urinary frequency at night

12

Drugs for Cardiovascular Diseases

Reading Drug Labels and Medication Orders

1. You receive the following prescription, and the drug label shown is the product you pick up from the pharmacy shelf:

   ℞   Catapres patch 0.2 mg q7 d

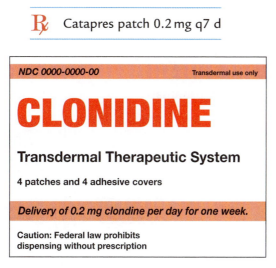

NDC 0000-0000-00   Transdermal use only

CLONIDINE

Transdermal Therapeutic System

4 patches and 4 adhesive covers

Delivery of 0.2 mg clondine per day for one week.

Caution: Federal law prohibits dispensing without prescription

   a. How many 0.2 mg patches will the patient receive for a one-month supply? Show your calculations.

   _____

   b. A box of Catapres has been opened. You want to confirm that no contents have been removed. What comes in a box of Catapres?

   _____

   _____

Name _____   Date _____

2. You receive the following prescription, and the available drug contains 4 g of resin in 9 g of powder:

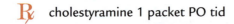

R̥ cholestyramine 1 packet PO tid

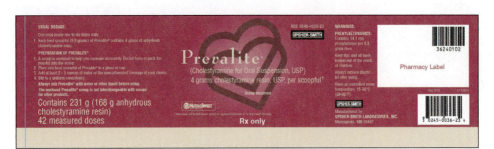

a. How many grams would the patient receive in one day?

_____

b. How should this product be prepared before administration?

_____

3. You receive the following order, and the drug label shown is the product you pick up from the pharmacy shelf:

R̥ amiodarone 900 mg/500 ml IV per atrial arrhythmia protocol

How many milliliters of amiodarone would you require to make this product?

_____

_____

4. You receive the following order:

R̥ metoprolol 400 mg PO daily

Based on the indicated dosing, what brand name version of metoprolol will need to be dispensed?

_____

5. You receive the following prescription:

> $\mathbf{R}$ Hyzaar 50/12.5 1 tab PO daily

a. What are the generic ingredients in this product?

_____

b. How many milligrams of diuretic will the patient receive in one month?

_____

6. You receive the following prescription, and the drug is available as a 20 mg/mL injection:

> $\mathbf{R}$ hydralazine 20 mg IV q6 h

The hospital requires a five-day supply to be stored in an automated dispensing machine on the floor. How many vials would you send to the floor? Show your calculations.

_____

_____

7. You receive the following prescription:

> $\mathbf{R}$ Lovenox (enoxaparin) 90 mg SC bid

Lovenox comes in the following syringes: 60 mg/0.6 mL, 80 mg/0.8 mL, 100 mg/mL, and 120 mg/0.8 mL
a. Which product would you select to fill this prescription?

_____

b. How many milliliters would correspond to the 90 mg dose?

_____

8. You receive the following prescription:

> $\mathbf{R}$ aspirin EC 325 mg PO daily

a. Why would enteric-coated (EC) aspirin be requested?

_____

b. How would this differ from a prescription for baby aspirin?

_____

9. You are assembling some pharmacy kits for the intensive care units at your hospital. The kit contains:

   #1 125 mg/25 mL vial of diltiazem for injection

   #1 100 mL bag of sodium chloride

   a. If these two products were added together, what would the resultant concentration be?

   _____

   b. If diltiazem is to be infused at a rate of 5 mg/hr, how long will it take to infuse 125 mg?

   _____

Understanding the Larger Medical Context

10. What does ACE and ARB stand for? In what ways is an ACE and an ARB different?

    _____

    _____

    _____

    _____

    _____

11. What is the major side effect of clopidogrel?

    _____

12. Why is Coreg given with food?

    _____

13. What drug classes are used for dyslipidemia?

    _____

    _____

14. How is nebivolol (Bystolic) different from other beta blockers?

    _____

    _____

15. Which lipoproteins are thought of as "good" cholesterol?

    _____

16. Which lipoproteins are thought of as "bad" cholesterol?

    _____

17. Why is it difficult to determine which size to dispense of the low-molecular-weight heparins? What should a pharmacy technician do before the product is dispensed?

_____

_____

_____

_____

_____

_____

18. The pharmacist suspects that a patient is having a heart attack and tells you to quickly get an aspirin. Would you get an 81 mg or a 325 mg aspirin? Would you get an enteric coated aspirin or a plain aspirin, and why?

_____

_____

19. Manufacturers are combining more than one drug into a tablet, especially heart and cholesterol medications. What are two reasons for combining drugs?

_____

Dispensing and Storing Drugs

Mark whether or not each of the following drugs must be dispensed in its original container.

20. Aggrenox   yes _____   no _____

21. Nitro Stat   yes _____   no _____

22. Plavix   yes _____   no _____

23. Edarbi   yes _____   no _____

24. lisinopril   yes _____   no _____

25. Nitro Dur   yes _____   no _____

26. Catapres patch   yes _____   no _____

27. digoxin tablets   yes _____   no _____

28. Lovenox syringes   yes _____   no _____

29. aspirin   yes _____   no _____

30. Lipitor tablets   yes _____   no _____

31. nifedipine XL   yes _____   no _____

32. Tekturna   yes _____   no _____

33. TriCor   yes _____   no _____

34. warfarin   yes _____   no _____

Which drugs have a black box warning (BBW), require a medication guide (MG), both (B), or neither (N)?

35. nadolol _____

36. Norvasc _____

37. amiodarone _____

38. Tikosyn _____

39. Multaq _____

40. digoxin _____

41. Lovenox _____

42. Asclera _____

43. Xarelto _____

44. Trilipix _____

45. Questran _____

46. Dilantin _____

47. aspirin _____

48. Coumadin _____

49. Valsartan _____

50. minoxidil _____

51. heparin _____

52. dabigatran _____

53. Crestor _____

54. dipyridamole _____

Putting Safety First

55. Which anticoagulants must have medication guides?

   _____

56. Which vasodilators have black box warnings?

   _____

57. Which cholesterol medication has a medication guide?

   _____

Does the dose match the medication? If not, give a common dose.

58. simvastatin 100

   _____

59. aspirin 10 g

   _____

Understanding Concepts

60. A clonidine patch should be worn for _____.

61. _____ is a fibrinolytic agent given in two injections of 10 mL separated by an interval of 30 minutes.

62. _____ is a membrane stabilizing agent that is also an anticonvulsant.

63. Dalteparin is an example of a low-molecular weight _____.

64. _____ pectoris is chest pain.

65. _____ is a waxlike constituent of animal origin that is important in discussion of circulatory health.

66. _____ stands for myocardial infarction, or heart attack.

67. _____ are a type of fat molecules that release fatty acids into the blood.

68. HF stands for _____.

69. An _____ is a variation from normal heart beat.

70. _____ is a slow heart rate.

71. _____ blood pressure is blood pressure during heart dilation.

72. A _____ is clotting within a blood vessel.

73. _____ is also known as a statin.

74. List the advantages of LMWHs over heparin.

   _____

   _____

   _____

   _____

Matching–Drug Names and Drug Groups

_____ 75. alfuzosin

_____ 76. amlodipine-atorvastatin

_____ 77. amlodipine-benazepril

_____ 78. amlodipine-valsartan

_____ 79. aspirin

_____ 80. aspirin-dipyridamole

_____ 81. atorvastatin

_____ 82. benazepril-hydrochlorothiazide

_____ 83. carvedilol

_____ 84. clonidine

_____ 85. clopidogrel

_____ 86. diltiazem

_____ 87. digoxin

_____ 88. ezetimibe

_____ 89. irbesartan

_____ 90. irbesartan-hydrochlorothiazide

_____ 91. losartan

_____ 92. losartan-hydrochlorothiazide

_____ 93. nisoldipine

_____ 94. olmesartan

_____ 95. phenytoin

_____ 96. pravastatin

_____ 97. propranolol

_____ 98. ramipril

_____ 99. rosuvastatin

_____ 100. simvastatin

_____ 101. telmisartan

_____ 102. trandolapril-verapamil

_____ 103. valsartan

_____ 104. valsartan-hydrochlorothiazide

_____ 105. warfarin

a. Aggrenox

b. Altace

c. Avalide

d. Avapro

e. Benicar

f. Caduet

g. Cardizem

h. Catapres

i. Coreg

j. Coumadin

k. Cozaar

l. Crestor

m. Dilantin

n. Diovan

o. Diovan HCT

p. Exforge

q. Hyzaar

r. Inderal

s. Lanoxin

t. Lipitor

u. Lotensin HCT

v. Lotrel

w. Micardis

x. Plavix

y. Pravachol

z. many names

aa. Sular

bb. Tarka

cc. Uroxatral

dd. Zetia

ee. Zocor

Matching–Terms and Definitions

_____ 106. angina pectoris

_____ 107. anticoagulant

_____ 108. antiplatelet

_____ 109. arrhythmia

_____ 110. beta blocker

_____ 111. bradycardia

_____ 112. calcium channel blocker

_____ 113. clotting cascade

_____ 114. heart failure (HF)

_____ 115. fibrinolytic

_____ 116. high-density lipoproteins (HDLs)

_____ 117. hyperlipidemia

_____ 118. hypertension

_____ 119. international normalized ratio (INR)

_____ 120. low-density lipoproteins (LDLs)

_____ 121. membrane stabilizing agent

_____ 122. myocardial infarction (MI)

_____ 123. partial thromboplastin time (PTT)

_____ 124. statin

_____ 125. cerebrovascular accident

_____ 126. tachycardia

_____ 127. thrombus

_____ 128. thrombocytopenia

_____ 129. transient ischemic attack (TIA)

a. A class I antiarrhythmic drug that slows the movement of ions into cardiac cells, thus reducing the action potential and dampening abnormal rhythms and heartbeats

b. A class II antiarrhythmic drug that competitively blocks response to beta adrenergic stimulation and therefore lowers heart rate, myocardial contractility, blood pressure, and myocardial oxygen demand; used to treat arrhythmias, MIs, and angina

c. A class IV antiarrhythmic drug that prevents the movement of calcium ions through slow channels; used for most supraventricular tachyarrhythmias and in angina

d. A condition in which the heart can no longer pump adequate blood to the body's tissues; results in engorgement of the pulmonary vessels

e. A decrease in the bone marrow production of blood platelets

f. A drug that prevents clot formation by affecting clotting factors

g. A drug that reduces the risk of clot formation by inhibiting platelet aggregation

h. A heart attack occurs when a region of the heart muscle is deprived of oxygen

i. A method of standardizing the prothrombin time (PT) by comparing it to a standard index

j. A series of events that initiate blood clotting, or coagulation

k. A test that measures the function of the intrinsic and common pathways in blood clotting; affected by heparin

l. Abnormally slow heart rate (below 60 beats per minute)

m. An agent that dissolves clots

n. An HMG-CoA reductase inhibitor, a drug that inhibits the rate-limiting step in cholesterol formation

o. Any variation from the normal heartbeat

p. Blood clot

q. Elevated blood pressure, where systolic blood pressure is greater than 140 mm Hg and diastolic pressure is greater than 90 mm Hg

r. Elevation of the levels of one or more of the lipoproteins in the blood

s. Excessively fast heart rate

t. Lipoproteins containing 5% triglyceride, 25% cholesterol, and 50% protein; "good cholesterol"

Definitions continued next page

u. Lipoproteins containing 6% triglycerides and 65% cholesterol; "bad cholesterol"

v. The result of an event (finite, ongoing, or protracted occurrences) that interrupts oxygen supply to an area of the brain; usually caused by cerebral infarction or cerebral hemorrhage

w. Spasmodic or suffocating chest pain caused by an imbalance between oxygen supply and oxygen demand

x. Temporary neurologic change that occurs when part of the brain lacks sufficient blood supply over a brief period of time; may be a warning sign and predictor of imminent cerebrovascular accident

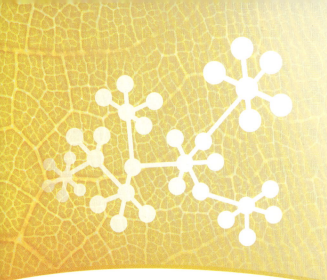

13

Drugs for Muscle and Joint Disease

Reading Drug and Medication Orders

1. You receive the following prescription, and the drug label shown is the product you pick up from the pharmacy shelf:

   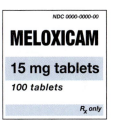

   NDC 0000-0000-00
   MELOXICAM
   15 mg tablets
   100 tablets
   R_x only

   ℞   Mobic 7.5 mg 1 po bid

   a. Is a medication guide required when the prescription is dispensed to the patient? Explain your answer.

   _____

   b. How many tablets are needed for a 30 day supply?

   _____

2. You receive the following prescription:

   ℞   Enbrel 50 mg SC weekly

   a. What is the drug class of Enbrel?

   _____

   b. When would a physician prescribe Enbrel for a patient?

   _____

   _____

Name _____ Date _____

3. You receive the following prescription:

> **R̶x̶** Ibuprofen 200 mg I-IV po daily prn pain

    a. Is this prescription Rx or OTC?

    _____

    b. How does ibuprofen work on pain?

    _____

4. What is the maximum daily dose of acetaminophen?

_____

Understanding the Larger Medical Context

5. What is a muscle, and what is a joint?

_____

_____

6. What are the advantages of using nonnarcotic analgesics compared to narcotic analgesics?

_____

_____

_____

7. What is a muscle relaxant, and what are the possible side effects of taking a muscle relaxant?

_____

_____

8. In what ways is osteoarthritis different from rheumatoid arthritis?

_____

_____

_____

_____

9. What role do cyclooxygenase-1 and cyclooxygenase-2 play in pain and inflammation?

_____

_____

10. How do nonsteroidal anti-inflammatory agents work?

_____

_____

_____

11. How do NSAIDs and opiates differ?

_____

_____

_____

_____

12. What are advantages and disadvantages of using DMARDs?

_____

_____

_____

_____

13. What is gout, and how does it affect the body?

_____

_____

_____

_____

14. What is the most common effect of NSAIDs, and how is it minimized?

_____

_____

15. What is a mixed analgesic?

_____

16. What is the antidote for an acetaminophen overdose?

_____

17. What is the only COX-2 still on the market?

_____

18. List five tips for patients using an NSAID.

_____

_____

_____

19. Which NSAIDs have parenteral forms?

_____

20. Which NSAIDs are available OTC?

_____

Dispensing and Storing Drugs

21. What auxiliary label would you put on all of the NSAIDs?

_____

22. What are contraindications to celecoxib use?

_____

23. What are infliximab's black box warnings?

_____

24. There is one class of drugs in this chapter for which every drug has a medication guide. Which class is it?

_____

Putting Safety First

25. Other than NSAIDs, which drug is used for acute gout attacks?

_____

26. What is the maximum asprin dose for an adult?

_____

27. Why must the prescriber be notified if a patient brings in a prescription for Tylenol with a dosage of more than 4 grams per day?

_____

_____

Understanding Concepts

28. _____ is the only NSAID available as a suppository.

29. Allopurinol and colchicine are prescribed to treat _____.

30. _____ is an NSAID that comes in patch form.

31. _____ was the first OTC analgesic for children since acetaminophen was approved.

32. _____ is the brand name for the COX-2 inhibitor.

33. _____ and _____ are both brand names for ibuprofen.

34. ACh is the abbreviation for _____, a neurotransmitter important in muscle contraction.

35. _____ arthritis is an autoimmune disease.

36. _____ syndrome is a condition most common in children exposed to chickenpox.

37. _____ pain originates in the organs and is sharp and stabbing.

38. _____ is a deposit of sodium urate at the joint.

39. _____ pain is dull and throbbing and originates from skin, muscle, or bone.

40. _____ is inflammation of the joints.

41. _____ is a painful condition in which muscles are in a state of continuous contraction.

42. _____ arthritis is the result of improper excretion of uric acid.

Matching–Drug Names and Drug Groups

_____ 43. acetaminophen

_____ 44. allopurinol

_____ 45. carisoprodol

_____ 46. celecoxib

_____ 47. cyclobenzaprine

_____ 48. diclofenac

_____ 49. esomeprazole-naproxen

_____ 50. ibuprofen

_____ 51. meloxicam

_____ 52. metaxalone

_____ 53. naproxen

a. Aleve

b. Celebrex

c. Flexeril

d. Mobic

e. Motrin

f. Skelaxin

g. Soma

h. Tylenol

i. Vimovo

j. Voltaren

k. Zyloprim

Matching–Terms and Definitions

_____ 54. analgesic

_____ 55. antipyretic

_____ 56. APAP

_____ 57. arthritis

_____ 58. ASA

_____ 59. autoimmune disease

_____ 60. Celebrex

_____ 61. cyclooxygenase-2 (COX-2)

_____ 62. disease-modifying antirheumatic drugs (DMARDs)

_____ 63. gouty arthritis

_____ 64. muscle relaxant

_____ 65. muscle spasticity

_____ 66. nonnarcotic analgesic

_____ 67. nonsteroidal anti-inflammatory drugs (NSAIDs)

_____ 68. osteoarthritis

_____ 69. rheumatoid arthritis

_____ 70. salicylates

_____ 71. SLE

a. A class of nonnarcotic analgesics that have both pain-relieving and antipyretic (fever reducing) properties

b. Degenerative joint disease resulting in loss of cartilage, elasticity, and thickness

c. An autoimmune disease in which the body's immune system attacks its own connective tissue; characterized by inflammation of the synovial membrane of the joints

d. A condition whereby muscle fibers are in a state of involuntary, continuous contraction that causes pain

e. A disease resulting from the improper excretion of uric acid; also called gout

f. A drug that reduces or prevents skeletal muscle contraction

g. A drug used for pain, inflammation, and fever that is not a controlled substance

h. An enzyme that is present in the synovial fluid of arthritis patients and is associated with the pain and inflammation of arthritis

i. Agents that can modify the progression of rheumatoid arthritis

j. Fever reducing

k. Illness in which the immune system attacks and destroys healthy tissue within the body

l. Joint inflammation; persistent pain due to functional problems of the joints

m. Anti-inflammatory, analgesic, and antipyretic drugs that are not controlled substances or steroids; used to treat arthritis and for other indications such as pain and inflammation

n. Pain relieving

o. aspirin

p. acetaminophen

q. Systemic Lupus Erythematosus

r. only Cox-2 inhibitor on market

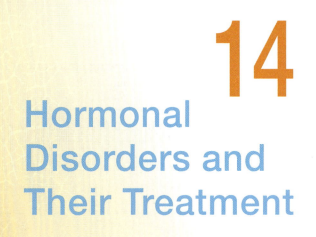

14

Hormonal Disorders and Their Treatment

Reading Drug Labels and Medication Orders

1. You receive the following prescription, and the drug label shown is the product you pick up from the pharmacy shelf:

℞   Medrol dose pack #1 as directed

NDC 0000-0000-00
21 Tablets
6505-01-131-5619

methylprednisolone tablets, USP

4 mg
Unit of Use

℞ only

See package
insert for
complete
product
information.

Keep patient under close observation of a physician.
Store at controlled room temperature
20° to 25°C (68° to 77°F) [see USP].

What are the instructions for a Medrol dose pack?

_____

_____

_____

Name _____ Date _____

2. You receive the following prescription, and the drug label shown is the product you pick up from the pharmacy shelf:

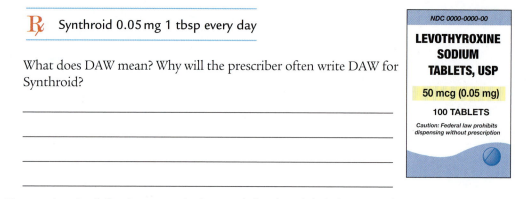

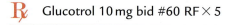
Synthroid 0.05 mg 1 tbsp every day

What does DAW mean? Why will the prescriber often write DAW for Synthroid?

_____

_____

_____

_____

3. You receive the following prescription, and the drug label shown is the product you pick up from the pharmacy shelf:

R̶x̶ Glucotrol 10 mg bid #60 RF × 5

a. Does the drug label correspond to the product indicated in the prescription? Explain your answer.

_____

_____

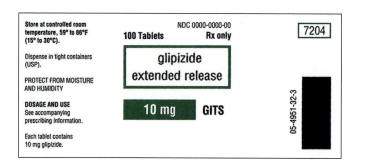

b. What is the drug class of Glucotrol, and for what medical condition is Glucotrol typically used? Explain the response the body has to Glucotrol.

_____

_____

c. What are the side effects of Glucotrol?

_____

_____

_____

4. You receive the following prescription for a 14-year-old patient who weighs exactly 44 kg. The drug label shown is the product to be dispensed, and you are to dispense the 12 mg cartridge.

℞   Humatrope 0.35 mg/kg weekly, given in daily SC INJ

a. What is the total weekly dose? Show your calculations.

_____

_____

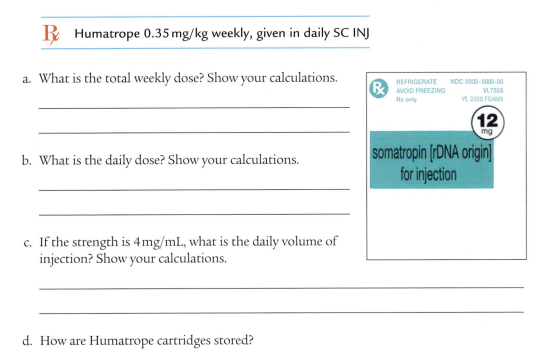

b. What is the daily dose? Show your calculations.

_____

_____

c. If the strength is 4 mg/mL, what is the daily volume of injection? Show your calculations.

_____

_____

d. How are Humatrope cartridges stored?

_____

_____

Understanding the Larger Medical Context

5. Explain the importance of exercising caution when using beta blockers in diabetic patients. Then list five signs and symptoms of hypoglycemia.

_____

_____

_____

_____

_____

_____

_____

_____

6. Name the four types of diabetes and identify the characteristics of each type.

_____

_____

_____

_____

_____

_____

_____

_____

7. What can cause hypothyroidism?

_____

_____

_____

_____

8. What are some causes of erectile dysfunction that are not related to medication?

_____

_____

9. What causes menopause to occur? When does menopause begin for women? What are common symptoms experienced by women during menopause?

_____

_____

_____

_____

10. What might cause a potential false-negative and a potential false-positive in a home pregnancy test?

_____

_____

_____

_____

_____

11. In what ways are osteoclasts and osteoblasts different?

_____

_____

_____

12. Describe the disorder discussed in this chapter that is primarily treated with corticosteroids. What are symptoms of this disorder?

_____

_____

_____

13. Describe the actions of insulin in the body.

_____

_____

14. What are the signs and symptoms of hyperthyroidism?

_____

_____

_____

_____

Dispensing and Storing Drugs

Where would the following medications be stored in the pharmacy?

15. Lantus

_____

16. Prolia

_____

17. Byetta

_____

Which of these drugs must have a medication guide?

18. Fosamax 10 mg   yes _____   no _____

19. Synthroid   yes _____   no _____

20. AndroGel   yes _____   no _____

21. Metformin   yes _____   no _____

22. Why is it important that women on oral contraceptives not smoke?

_____

_____

_____

23. What is the drug schedule of testosterone substances?

_____

24. What does DAW mean?

_____

_____

25. Why is it important to make sure the pharmacist counsels the patient when he or she gets a steroid dose pack? How are dose packs different from other medications? Can the technician counsel the patient if the pharmacist is busy?

_____

_____

_____

Putting Safety First

26. Which drug for erectile dysfunction requires a medication guide?

_____

27. Which insulins are available in concentrations higher than 100 units/mL? What concentration are they available in?

_____

28. Why is selecting the correct insulin concentration important?

_____

29. Femring is supplied on a ring inserted into the vagina for how long?

_____

30. How often is alendronate dosed?

_____

Understanding Concepts

31. _____ is usually the initial drug therapy for type 2 diabetes.

32. _____ is an agent used for diabetic ulcers.

33. _____ is a generic drug indicated for the treatment and prevention of osteoporosis in post-menopausal women and in Paget's bone disease for both men and women.

34. _____ is the inhaled insulin product.

35. _____ is a male hormone that is manufactured as a buccal system.

36. _____ is referred to as the "weekender" because it is effective for 36 hours.

37. _____ is the generic name of the erectile dysfunction drug that can be injected or inserted as a urethral pellet.

38. _____ generics are the actual brand name oral contraceptives relabeled and marketed under a generic product name, not listed in the orange book.

39. _____ is conjugated estrogen made from a pregnant mare's urine.

40. _____ is a combination of glyburide and metformin.

41. Women who are taking biphosphanates for bone loss should also be taking calcium and _____.

42. Technicians must make sure the pharmacist counsels anyone taking oral contraceptives and an _____, because the oral contraceptive becomes less effective when that type of drug is added.

43. An _____ is a cell that forms bone.

44. _____ is the gland that produces hormones that stimulate various body tissues.

45. _____ oral contraceptive regimens change doses once during the menstrual cycle.

46. _____ stands for pelvic inflammatory disease.

47. _____ and _____ are the most common side effects of emergency contraception.

48. _____ is the brand name for _____, a transdermal contraceptive.

49. List two reasons for hormone replacement in menopausal women: _____

_____

Matching–Drug Names and Drug Groups

_____ 50. alendronate

_____ 51. conjugated estrogen

_____ 52. estradiol

_____ 53. estradiol-levonorgestrel

_____ 54. ethinyl estradiol-levonorgestrel

_____ 55. ethinyl estradiol–norgestimate

_____ 56. ethinyl estradiol-norelgestromin

_____ 57. glimepiride

_____ 58. glipizide

_____ 59. glyburide

_____ 60. insulin glargine

_____ 61. insulin lispro

_____ 62. levothyroxine

_____ 63. methylprednisolone

_____ 64. risedronate

_____ 65. sildenafil

_____ 66. tadalafil

a. Actonel

b. Amaryl

c. Aviane

d. Cialis

e. Climara Pro

f. Fosamax

g. Glucotrol

h. Humalog

i. Lantus

j. Micronase

k. Ortho Evra

l. Ortho Tri-Cyclen

m. Premarin

n. Solu-Medrol

o. Synthroid

p. Viagra

q. Vivelle Dot

Matching–Terms and Definitions

_____ 67. AB rated

_____ 68. DAW

_____ 69. estrogen

_____ 70. gestational diabetes

_____ 71. glucocorticoid

_____ 72. HbA1C

_____ 73. erectile dysfunction

_____ 74. oral contraceptive (OCs)

_____ 75. osteoporosis

_____ 76. progesterone

_____ 77. testosterone

_____ 78. virilization

a. A combination of one or more hormonal compounds taken orally to prevent the occurrence of pregnancy

b. A hormone that is responsible for sperm production, sexual potency, and the maintenance of muscle mass and strength, among other functions

c. Corticosteroid involved in metabolism and immune system regulation

d. Diabetes that occurs during pregnancy when insufficient insulin is produced

e. Failure of the male to initiate or to maintain an erection until ejaculation

f. Glycosylated hemoglobin; an "average" of the sugar measured in blood glucose over a period of time

g. Instruction in a prescription to prevent substitution of generic drugs for the branded drug

h. Refers to a generic drug rated as bioequivalent to the branded drug by the FDA as shown by an experimental study

i. One of the group of hormones that stimulate the growth of reproductive tissue in females

j. The condition of reduced bone mineral density, disrupted microarchitecture of bone structure, and increased likelihood of fracture

k. The development of male characteristics

l. The hormone that prepares the uterus for the reception and development of the fertilized ovum

15

Topical, Ophthalmic, and Otic Medications

Reading Drug Labels and Medication Orders

1. You receive the following prescription:

   R℟ tretinoin cream 0.05% apply daily for wrinkles

   a. You identify Retin-A cream 0.05% as the product available. Is this the correct product? Explain your answer.

   _____

   _____

   _____

   b. How does tretinoin work?

   _____

   _____

   _____

2. While you are working in the pharmacy, a physician calls and asks you to send Bactroban ointment for treating a patient with impetigo. The physician mentions that the patient has multiple lesions. You have Bactroban cream in the pharmacy. Would you send this product? Explain your answer.

   _____

   _____

   _____

   _____

   _____

Name _____ **Date** _____

3. A patient brings in the following prescription and asks how to use it:

R_x Floxin Otic Instill 10 drops AU daily

How would a patient administer this product?

_____

_____

_____

Understanding the Larger Medical Context

4. When treating skin ailments, can creams and ointments be interchanged? What could result if the medications were interchanged on a dermatologist's prescription?

_____

_____

_____

_____

_____

5. What is acne? What causes acne?

_____

_____

_____

6. Is it common practice for the prescriber to write a prescription for an ophthalmic agent to be used in the ear? Is it common practice for an otic agent to be used in the eye? Explain your answers.

_____

_____

_____

7. In what ways are open-angle glaucoma and narrow-angle glaucoma different? Which type of glaucoma is more common?

_____

_____

_____

_____

_____

8. As a pharmacy technician, what can you do to help patients prevent photosensitivity?

_____

_____

_____

_____

_____

9. A patient recently started diphenhydramine for her allergies and developed sunburn while gardening outside. She wants your help in selecting a sunscreen because she does not understand what SPF, UV-A, or UV-B mean. How do you explain the differences among the notations?

_____

_____

_____

_____

_____

_____

_____

10. Write instructions for applying eye ointment in language a patient would understand.

_____

_____

_____

11. Are OTC medications to treat head lice as effective as a prescription medication? Explain your answer.

_____

_____

Dispensing and Storing Drugs

Which drugs require medication guides (MG), have black box warnings (BBW), both (B), or neither (N)?

12. Xalatan _____

13. Accutane _____

14. BenzaClin _____

15. erythromycin ophthalmic ointment _____

16. Protopic _____

17. Retin-A _____

18. Elidel _____

19. Ciprodex _____

20. Ciloxan _____

Putting Safety First

Does the indication match the drug? If not, list what the drug is commonly used for.

21. pyrethrins for ringworm

_____

22. Botox for wrinkles

_____

23. benzoyl peroxide wash for sunburn

_____

24. tretinoin for wrinkles

_____

25. azelaic acid for acne

_____

26. Efudex for narrow-angle glaucoma

_____

27. tacrolimus for eczema

_____

28. ivermectin for ear infections

_____

29. calamine for scabies

_____

30. nizoral for dandruff

_____

Understanding Concepts

31. Patients on ventilators who have scheduled mouth cleansings throughout the day with _____ have decreased incidences of pneumonia.

32. _____ is a prescription only product used for dandruff.

33. _____ and _____ are commonly used otic fluoroquinolones for otitis media.

34. _____ is a sunscreen with UVA-1, UVA-2, and UVB coverage.

35. _____ is a skin disorder characterized by patches of red, scaly, raised areas that usually occurs on elbows and knees.

36. Retin-A is approved only to treat_____ vulgaris but is used off label to diminish wrinkles.

37. The _____ is the layer of skin below the epidermis.

38. Vitreous _____ is fluid present in the eye.

39. Actinic _____ is a condition with scaly skin lesions that are pre-cancerous.

40. _____ is an ophthalmic disorder characterized by high internal eye pressure.

41. _____ is the top layer of skin.

42. Contact _____ is an inflammatory reaction produced by contact with an irritating agent.

43. _____ is the most serious form of malignant skin cancer.

44. _____ _____ , also known as eczema, produces chronic pruritic eruptions.

45. _____ is an abnormal response of the skin or eye to sunlight.

46. _____ is another term for pinkeye.

47. If a drug is _____, it will cause birth defects.

48. A _____ is a virally caused epidermal tumor.

49. _____, which stands for sun protection factor, is a rating given to sunscreens.

Matching–Brand and Generic Drug Names

_____ 50. clotrimazole

_____ 51. fluticasone

_____ 52. latanoprost

_____ 53. triamcinolone

_____ 54. tretinoin

_____ 55. acyclovir

_____ 56. metronidazole

_____ 57. azelaic acid

_____ 58. terbinafine

_____ 59. mupirocin

a. Cutivate

b. Kenalog

c. Alevazol

d. Xalatan

e. Bactroban

f. Zovirax

g. Azelex

h. Lamisil

i. Retin-A

j. MetroGel

Matching–Terms and Definitions

_____ 60. eczema

_____ 61. carbuncle

_____ 62. impetigo

_____ 63. keratolytic

_____ 64. pediculosis

_____ 65. photosensitivity

_____ 66. ringworm

a. A coalescent mass of infected hair follicles that is deeper than a furuncle

b. A fungus that infects the horny (scaly) layer of skin or the nails; also called tinea

c. A hot, itchy, red, oozing skin inflammation; also called dermatitis

d. A superficial, highly contagious skin infection; characterized by small red spots that evolve into vesicles, break, become encrusted, and are surrounded by a zone of erythema

e. An agent that breaks down and peels off dead skin cells to keep them from clogging pores

f. An abnormal response of the skin or eye to sunlight

g. An infestation of lice

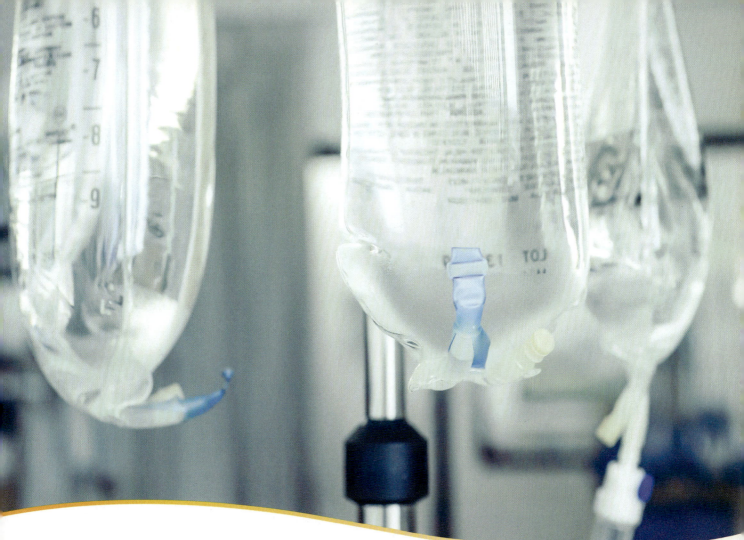

16

Cancer Drugs and Chemotherapy

Reading Drug Labels and Medication Orders

1. Mr. Kelly is currently being treated for colon cancer. Mr. Kelly is 47 years old, 70 inches tall, and weighs 215 lbs. He is starting FOLFOX-6 as his new regimen. The regimen details per cycle are as follows:

    Eloxatin 85 mg/m^2 on day 1

    leucovorin 400 mg/m^2 on day 1

    5-fluorouracil bolus 400 mg/m^2 on day 1

    5-fluorouracil continuous infusion 3,000 mg/m^2 over 46 hours on day 1 and day 2

    a. Find a BSA calculator online (your instructor will suggest some website options), and determine Mr. Kelly's BSA using the formula deleveped by DuBois and DuBois.

    _____

    b. The concentration for the 5-fluorouracil (5-FU) is 50 mg/mL. How many milliliters will the bolus be? Show your calculations.

    _____

    _____

    c. The following three facts about oxaliplatin are important to know:
    - During the FOLFOX-6 regimen, oxaliplatin must be given at the same time as leucovorin.
    - Oxaliplatin is not compatible with any solutions that contain sodium chloride.
    - Oxaliplatin is usually in a concentration of 3 mg/mL to 5 mg/mL.

    Based on these three facts, what would be an appropriate diluent and volume for the leucovorin?

    _____

Name _____ **Date** _____

d. How many vials of Eloxatin will be required for three cycles of therapy? Show your calculations.

_____

_____

e. The calculated dose for the 5-FU continuous infusion is 6,450 mg. If Mr. Kelly is set to receive this medication through an outpatient infusion pump at a rate of 3 mL/hour for the duration of the infusion, how many milliliters must be provided for the course of therapy?

_____

2. Mr. Kelly undergoes three cycles of therapy without improvement. The oncologist decides to add Erbitux to the treatment regimen at a dose of 400 mg/m^2. The drug label shows the drug to be dispensed.

a. What is Mr. Kelly's resulting dose?

_____

b. How many vials will be required per dose? Show your calculations.

_____

_____

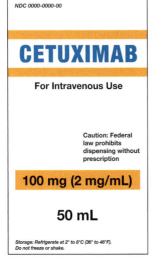

NDC 0000-0000-00

CETUXIMAB

For Intravenous Use

Caution: Federal law prohibits dispensing without prescription

100 mg (2 mg/mL)

50 mL

Storage: Refrigerate at 2° to 8°C (36° to 46°F). Do not freeze or shake.

3. Mrs. Baribeault is currently being treated with ABVD, a regimen with a high incidence of anemia. She has a hemoglobin of 9.6, which is being treated with Epogen with the following instructions.

℞   Epogen 40,000 units SC once a week

a. How many milliliters of Epogen will be required per dose?

_____

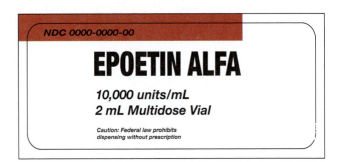

NDC 0000-0000-00

EPOETIN ALFA

10,000 units/mL
2 mL Multidose Vial

Caution: Federal law prohibits dispensing without prescription

b. How many vials of Epogen will be required per dose?

_____

4. Ms. Amik, a survivor of breast cancer, presents the following prescription:

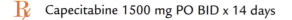

 R_x Capecitabine 1500 mg PO BID x 14 days

a. How many milligrams will Ms. Amik receive for this prescription?

_____

b. The pills in the pharmacy come in a 500 mg tablets. How would you write the instructions for the prescription label?

_____

5. Mr. Garza, a patient currently being treated for colon cancer, is being started on oxaliplatin.

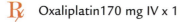

 R_x Oxaliplatin170 mg IV x 1

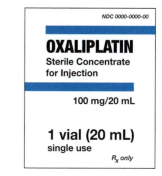

NDC 0000-0000-00

OXALIPLATIN
Sterile Concentrate
for Injection

100 mg/20 mL

1 vial (20 mL)
single use

R_x only

a. How many milliliters of oxaliplatin will be used for the product shown in the drug label?

_____

_____

b. What is a unique toxicity of oxaliplatin?

_____

_____

6. Mrs. Blanchard is being treated with carboplatin-paclitaxel for ovarian cancer. Her regimen is as follows. She is 65 inches tall and weighs 160 lbs.

 R_x Paraplatin AUC = 5

 Taxol 175 mg/m^2

Web

a. Using the calculator at **http://Pharmacology6e.ParadigmCollege.net/calculator**, what is the patient's BSA?

_____

b. If the concentration for the Taxol vial is 6 mg/mL, how many milliliters of Taxol will be used per dose? Show your calculations.

_____

_____

c. The pharmacist calculates the Paraplatin dose to be 500 mg. How many milliliters of Paraplatin must be used if the concentration is 10 mg/mL?

_____

Understanding the Larger Medical Context

7. Describe the cell kill hypothesis theory.

    _____

    _____

    _____

    _____

8. Describe the four major modalities for treating cancer.

    _____

    _____

9. Compare and contrast primary, adjuvant, and palliative chemotherapy.

    _____

    _____

10. Describe the target and benefits of using cell cycle-specific drugs.

    _____

    _____

Dispensing and Storing Drugs

11. List four possible methods of accidental exposure to chemotherapy agents.

    _____

    _____

    _____

    _____

    _____

12. When should personal protective equipment be used? What are examples of personal protective equipment?

    _____

    _____

    _____

13. If an accidental spill occurs, what should be referred to that guides the cleanup process?

    _____

14. List two inventory or storage measures to prevent the dispensing of chemotherapy in error.

    _____

    _____

Putting Safety First

Do the following orders match typical preventive measures for the listed drugs? If not, describe appropriate preventive measures.

15. Administer aggressive IV fluids after each dose of cisplatin.

    _____

    _____

16. Give mesna during and after dacarbazine treatment.

    _____

17. Administer steroid eyedrops during treatment whenever patients receive doses >1,000 mg/m2 of cytarabine.

    _____

    _____

18. Administer folic acid and vitamin B12 supplements, starting 5–7 days before treatment with pemetrexed.

    _____

    _____

19. Cap individual doses at 2 mg for irinotecan.

    _____

    _____

Understanding Concepts

20. _____, _____, and _____ are major side effects of antimetabolites.

21. Chlorambucil and melphalan belong to a group called the _____ agents.

22. MAB stands for _____.

23. _____ agents are a class of chemotherapy agents that bind to and damage DNA during the cell division process, ultimately preventing cell replication.

24. _____ alkaloids are derived from periwinkle plants and are used in treatments of various cancers.

25. _____ are antimicrotubule drugs that are derived from yew trees.

26. _____ is a chemotherapy agent derived from the American mayapple plant.

27. _____ work by blocking the activity of testosterone at the receptor level or interfering with the production of testosterone.

28. _____ should always be worn when working with hazardous drugs, even when delivering them to the site where they will be infused into the patient.

29. _____ _____ prevent formation of blood vessels that allow for tumor growth and invasion of surrounding tissue.

Matching–Drug Names and Drug Groups

_____ 30. axitinib

_____ 31. capecitabine

_____ 32. mercaptopurine

_____ 33. panitumumab

_____ 34. topotecan

_____ 35. trastuzumab

_____ 36. doxorubicin

_____ 37. sunitinib

_____ 38. sorafenib

_____ 39. fluorouracil

a. Hycamtin

b. Herceptin

c. Xeloda

d. Purinethol

e. Inlyta

f. Vectibix

g. Sutent

h. Adrucil

i. Adriamycin

j. Nexavar

Matching–Malignancy with Drug

_____ 40. bladder

_____ 41. colon

_____ 42. breast

_____ 43. rectal

_____ 44. leukemia

_____ 45. lung

_____ 46. lymphoma

_____ 47. melanoma

_____ 48. non-Hodgkins

_____ 49. multiple myeloma

_____ 50. prostate

_____ 51. ovarian

_____ 52. testicular

_____ 53. stomach

a. Alkeran (melphalan)

b. rituximab

c. Blenoxane (bleomycin)

d. bicalutamide

e. Vectibix (panitumumab)

f. Eloxatin (oxaliplatin)

g. Ellence (epirubicin)

h. Treanda (bendamustine)

i. Gemzar (gemcitabine)

j. Paraplatin (carboplatin)

k. Cytoxan (cyclophosphamide)

l. Taxol (paclitaxel)

m. Ifex (ifosfamide)

n. Temodar (temozolomide)

Matching–Terms and Definitions

_____ 54. antimetabolites

_____ 55. cytotoxic drugs

_____ 56. extravasation

_____ 57. metastasis

_____ 58. spill kits

_____ 59. immunotherapy

_____ 60. tumor burden

_____ 61. investigational drugs

_____ 62. melanoma

_____ 63. threshold dose

a. A drug used in clinical trials that has not yet been approved by the FDA for use in the general population, or a drug used for nonapproved indications

b. Equipment used where hazardous drugs are prepared, administered, or transported

c. The lifetime cumulative dose limit for a drug

d. The number of cancer cells or the size of the tumor tissue

e. A type of cancer treatment that stimulates the immune system to stop or slow the growth of cancer cells

f. The process of a tumor having spread from its primary site to other parts of the body

g. Drugs that interfere with some normal process of cell function or proliferation

h. Drugs that work in the synthesis phase of the cell cycle

i. A frequently fatal type of skin cancer

j. The escape of IV fluids into the surrounding tissue

17

Vitamins, Electrolytes, Nutrition, Antidotes, and Bioterrorism

Reading Drug Labels and Medication Orders

1. You receive the following prescription, and the drug label shown is the product you pick up from the pharmacy shelf:

℞ Cipro 500 mg i bid #120

a. Is this prescription okay to fill as written?

_____

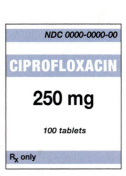

NDC 0000-0000-00

CIPROFLOXACIN

250 mg

100 tablets

℞ₓ only

b. Using the medication indicated in the drug label, how many tablets would you dispense to fill this prescription?

_____

_____

2. While working in the emergency room pharmacy, you receive a stat order. The physician needs an empiric dose for acute digoxin toxicity.

a. What products are available for treating digoxin overdose?

_____

_____

b. What is the empiric dose for acute digoxin toxicity?

_____

Name _____ Date _____

Understanding the Larger Medical Context

3. What is the difference between the calcium salts gluconate, chloride, carbonate, citrate, and acetate?

_____

_____

_____

_____

_____

_____

_____

4. What are the two types of total parenteral nutrition? How are they different?

_____

_____

_____

_____

_____

_____

_____

_____

5. What is the difference between fat-soluble and water-soluble vitamins? Name two examples of each type.

_____

_____

_____

6. When is a Code Blue initiated?

_____

_____

7. What are typical causes of water deficit?

_____

_____

8. Why is tonicity important when preparing IV fluids?

_____

_____

9. What is bioterrorism? Which agents have the potential to become biologic weapons?

_____

_____

_____

_____

_____

_____

_____

10. In the event of a biologic attack, what role would pharmacy technicians play?

_____

_____

11. The emergency room physician calls the pharmacy and tells you that the dobutamine solution in the Blue-Alert cart has turned a light pink color. The physician wants the solution replaced stat. What do you tell the physician about dobutamine?

_____

_____

_____

_____

_____

Dispensing and Storing Drugs

Are the following medications available over the counter or by prescription?

12. calcium acetate

_____

13. vitamin B_{12} 1000 mcg INJ

_____

14. etomidate

_____

15. activated charcoal

_____

16. vitamin K

_____

17. penicillamine

_____

18. pyridoxine

_____

19. vitamin D$_2$

_____

20. calcium gluconate

_____

21. Jevity Plus

_____

Putting Safety First

22. When mixing TPN, which elements have to be separated so they do not precipitate in the bag?

_____

_____

_____

_____

23. What is the purpose of epinephrine in a Code Blue emergency kit?

_____

_____

_____

_____

24. What are the three types of anthrax? How is anthrax treated?

_____

_____

25. What is ricin? What harm can it cause the human body?

_____

_____

26. What are the fat-soluble vitamins? Why is it important for people to limit the amount of over-the-counter fat-soluble vitamins they ingest?

_____

_____

Understanding Concepts

27. _____ are molecular compounds that form ions when dissolved in water.

28. _____ is known as a family of compounds referred to as retinoic acids.

29. _____ nitrite is an antidote for cyanide poisoning.

30. Activated _____ is a treatment in the emeregency room for cases of poisoning.

31. _____ is another name for tocopherol.

32. _____ is an antidote for spider bites.

33 _____ is an antidote for scorpion bites.

34. _____ is a name for vitamin B_1.

35. _____ is a name for vitamin B_2.

36. _____ is a vitamin that acts as a coenzyme in carbohydrate metabolism.

37. If a script is written for ergocalciferol, it is for vitamin _____.

38. _____ is a name for vitamin B_3.

39. _____ is a name for vitamin B_5.

40. _____ is a name for vitamin B_6.

41. _____ is a name for vitamin B_9.

42 _____ is a name for vitamin B_{12}.

43. _____ acid is vitamin B_9.

44. _____ acid is vitamin C.

45. A drug that counters the harmful effects of a poison is an _____.

46. _____ is a toxin derived from castor beans.

47. _____ is a condition caused by vitamin D deficiency.

48. When the lipid separates from the parental nutrition solution, this is referred to as _____.

49. Low blood pH is referred to as _____.

50. High blood pH is referred to as _____.

51. Code _____ is an institutional signal that a life-threatening situation is occurring.

Matching–Drug Names and Drug Groups

_____ 52. amiodarone

_____ 53. digoxin immune Fab

_____ 54. epinephrine

_____ 55. lorcaserin

_____ 56. fomepizole

_____ 57. naloxone

_____ 58. glucagon

_____ 59. potassium

_____ 60. pralidoxime

_____ 61. verapamil

a. Cordarone

b. Digibind

c. Klor Con

d. Narcan

e. Calan

f. Adrenalin

g. Belviq

h. GlucaGen

i. Protopam

j. Antizol

Matching–Terms and Definitions

_____ 62. antidote

_____ 63. antivenin

_____ 64. chelating agent

_____ 65. coenzyme

_____ 66. cracking

_____ 67. enteral nutrition

_____ 68. gastric lavage

_____ 69. isotonic solution

_____ 70. parenteral nutrition

_____ 71. pooling

_____ 72. probiotic

_____ 73. tocopherol

_____ 74. tonicity

_____ 75. vitamin

a. A procedure to wash out or irrigate the patient's stomach, commonly known as a stomach pump

b. Feeding a patient by supplying a nutrient solution through a vein

c. A drug that bonds to a metal ion to prevent it from reacting with biological compounds

d. A chemical other than a protein that is needed to assist an enzyme in performing a metabolic function

e. An organic substance that is necessary for the normal metabolic functioning of the body but that the body does not synthesize, so it must be obtained from food

f. Feeding a patient liquid food through a tube that leads to the gastrointestinal system

g. A drug that counters the harmful effects of a poison

h. A solution with the same level of particles, and thus the same tonicity, as body fluids

i. A material used in treatment of poisoning by animal venom

j. The relationship of a solution to the body's own fluids; measured by determining the number of dissolved particles in solution

k. One of the alcohols that constitute vitamin E

l. A product to restore or promote the growth of normal bacterial flora in the body

m. Separation of lipid from a parenteral nutrition solution

n. A time-saving process used when preparing a three-in-one TPN, in which all electrolytes except phosphate are put into a small-volume parenteral bag and then transferred into each batch

Notes